MY BEAUTIFUL PSYCHOSIS

MY BEAUTIFUL PSYCHOSIS
Making Sense of Madness

Emma Goude

AEON

First published in 2020 by
Aeon Books
PO Box 76401
London W5 9RG

British Library Cataloguing in Publication Data

A C.I.P. for this book is available from the British Library

ISBN-13: 978-1-91280-795-6

Typeset by Medlar Publishing Solutions Pvt Ltd, India
Printed in Great Britain

www.aeonbooks.co.uk

Cover artwork *Straight Jacket* by Adriane Vinter

Grateful acknowledgement is made to the following for permissions to use material: Si John and Jennifer Berezan www.edgeofwonder.com

Some names of persons in this book have been changed.

This book is not intended as a substitute for the medical advice of a physician. The reader should regularly consult a physician in matters relating to his/her health and particularly with respect to any symptoms that may require diagnosis or medical attention.

For
Daniel Kilroy, one of many,
who didn't make it.

'When a flower doesn't bloom, you fix the environment in which it grows, not the flower.'

—Alexander Den Heijer

CONTENTS

EPISODE FIVE

EPISODE SIX

EPISODE SEVEN

FOREWORD

I first met Emma on the Open Dialogue training. She had agreed to film the first couple of years of our training and I had heard that she had her own previous lived experience but I knew little more. I got to know her during the course of the training, however, and it was clear that she was supportive of the change we have been trying to bring about. What I didn't appreciate, though, was the depth and degree of passion with which she felt this. And then one day it became clear.

In the middle of something we call a fish bowl—where students take turns at sitting in a circle and sharing their feelings with one another— Emma joined us. It was the end of an intense week and there was a lot of emotion in the room, but in the end, Emma was the one who moved us most. She told us about how much of her time behind the camera had been spent in tears. So much of the pain in the system that we had been reflecting on resonated with her and her own life. It was as a result of this that she felt deeply that change was needed, and she implored us to stay the course. Change wasn't going to be easy but she assured us that it was desperately needed. Many of us shed a tear hearing Emma's powerful words that day. She enabled us to leave inspired that we were on the right track. Ultimately her words served an important function in that first year of the first ever Open Dialogue training in the UK, and that was to remind us of just how much was at stake and just how much this change meant to people.

The role of champion for change is one that Emma has now taken to a new level. Amid all the training and research and organisational shift that's needed to really make a difference, the most important thing has to be the profoundly moving stories that lie at the heart of it all. And Emma's is exactly such a story.

I didn't know much of the detail of her story before I started to read this book and I certainly didn't know anything about her talent as a writer. From the first page, however, I was hooked. The sheer ambition of what she has attempted is easy to underestimate. To really convey the richness of a human story of someone who has been through the myriad twists and turns, the highs and lows that she has, requires real skill. And yet Emma transports us wholesale into her life. We feel as if we are travelling her path alongside her and repeatedly we are lifted then dropped and then lifted again along the way. Before this book I would not have believed it was possible to convey the true depth of the kind of experience Emma has had, but now I know otherwise.

Emma's is a journey that many of us need to travel to really understand what it is like to be in her shoes. Professionals can benefit deeply from the lens Emma brings to our work, and others with lived experience can also find genuine avenues for growth and hope in her inspiring words.

Emma, I think, correctly identifies that this is a time of great change. Something is shifting about the way we view and respond to mental distress. There is an increasing understanding of the need to listen to rather than shun the voices that emerge from such experiences. Indeed, in other cultures it is exactly these voices that are heard with the most reverence. And given the trajectory that our own civilisation seems to be taking right now, we could well benefit from different approaches and world views than our current one.

At the end of another training week, towards the end of Emma's time filming our course, Emma chose to sing a song for us. It's often a time of merriment and celebration as a course draws to a close, but as Emma began to sing we all fell silent. She played a small keyboard and softly sang the Tears for Fears song, 'Mad World'. It was a message that resonated with us all in that moment. Many shed tears again that night. There is indeed much that is mad about the way we organise our society today, and perhaps it is those who we lock up—physically or metaphorically—or marginalise or stigmatise that are, in many respects, the sane ones.

The powerful, inspiring and raw honesty of this book is truly a case in point. Often the most silenced voices are the ones that most need to be heard. My hope is that Emma's will now be.

Dr Russell Razzaque
London
March 2019

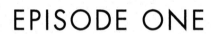

EPISODE ONE

CHAPTER ONE

Dope

The way Solomon scoops out the avocado with his hands is so erotic I don't know what to do with myself. It's so obvious where this is going; why can't I just let myself go with it? I'm frozen with excruciating self-consciousness. An invisible straitjacket shackles me. Does he realise how sexual it is or is he just innocently enjoying the sensuousness of the olive green flesh? I admire how he just gets right in and makes a big mess. I would have used some kind of utensil, efficient and clean but not nearly as pleasurable. Pleasure, that's it. He's immersed in the pleasure of how the fruit feels in his hands.

'It's so ripe,' he smiles at me raising a single eyebrow, then licks the creamy flesh off his fingers. Not knowing where to put myself, I sit down at the kitchen table and decide to play it cool. It's just an avocado.

His flatmate, Nat, arrives home and takes the seat opposite me. I've met Nat a few times before and he seems fun.

'Hi,' I say, a little too keen perhaps, but grateful for the interruption to the sexually charged meal preparations. 'We're just about to have dinner. You're very welcome to join us.' I'm trying to say, *hey, I'm not going to steal your friend away from you.*

I like Nat. When I first met him, I overheard him say to Sol, 'Your new girlfriend's *hot*.' I'm not sure we're boyfriend and girlfriend because we don't really talk about that but it was good to hear Nat giving me the thumbs up. It's not my place to invite him to join us for dinner, but I feel less awkward with him here. Solomon doesn't object but I can tell he's not happy about it. He's nice enough to me but he keeps snapping at Nat.

Once we've finished eating, Nat heads off, leaving me alone again with Solomon. Sol puts some music on and I roll a joint for something to do. I'm feeling a little more comfortable now we've eaten and sex isn't so obviously on the menu. I take a drag, hold my breath for a couple of seconds, and blow out the remnants. My heart feels jittery in my chest. *Maybe dope wasn't such a good idea*, I think, passing Sol the spliff.

'Cheers, Em,' he says. I like the way he says Em. It feels familiar.

'Sorry I invited your flatmate. I was just trying to be nice,' I explain.

'He had a bit of a cheek,' Sol blurts. 'Gooseberrying.' He pauses and reels himself in a bit. 'Maybe I was a bit passive-aggressive.' I don't know what to say. He was definitely passive-aggressive.

We're both silent for a while, letting the conversation find a new tack. I notice the music filling the gap created by our quietness. Sol stands up and kicks his leg out behind him, dancing to the drum and bass. He's mocking a little, maybe out of shyness, but I think he looks pretty cool. His number one haircut, covering up his receding hairline—like Bruce Willis—makes him look ultra-sexy. I always wondered how you're supposed to dance to drum and bass. Hopping to the drum and kicking to the bass, Solomon makes it look easy. He smiles at me, a cute smile, and I giggle nervously back.

'Brrrrat booooom,' he mimics the beats. I laugh and get up to join him, hopping on my right leg as I kick my left leg out behind me, arms poised like a runner about to start a race. We both swap legs at the same time. I seem to have picked it up quicker than I thought. Thank God I can dance.

It's tiring doing this stoned but it feels good, and it has lifted the mood. I can't keep it up for long, though, so I slow it down, picking out the bass rhythm. The track moves into a darker techno phase and I follow it, letting my body go with the music, the chaos snapping me out of my straitjacket.

We turn to face each other and smile, still dancing. I don't feel awkward any more. I'm lost in the musical vibes, and in my jerky movements. Sol turns around, wiggling his butt. I make a turn, shimmying around on the spot and shaking my arse in response. We both spin around at the same time and instead of returning full circle, we stop half way, wiggling our bums together. We close the gap between us, our backs finding each other. I feel his movement through my spine and sync my moves to his. The music shifts down a gear into a jazzier feel and we sway, each supporting the other.

Solomon bends forwards and I follow him, arching backwards. I feel the strength of his legs beneath him holding us both up, so I rest my weight on his. My feet are off the ground now and we're perfectly balanced. He judders his knees to the music, bouncing me up and down, my whole body limp on his back, arms dangling by my sides. His jiggling goes right through me, shaking loose any residual tension, every movement a massage. Something tugs in my hips, pulling my awareness down. Sol keeps a rhythm of short, sharp bumps to the beat. Inside I'm tingling, tiny bubbles making their way to the surface and popping through my skin. Shivers ripple outwards and down my legs, my cells giving a standing ovation.

Sol straightens up slowly and walks around to face me.

'Oh my God.' I grasp my head in my hands waiting for my vision to return. Sol giggles, pleased with my reaction. He takes my hand and leads me into the bedroom.

* * *

They sit opposite me at a desk that's now facing mine. We've been told to rearrange the office, make it more conducive to working together, instead of in our separate little competitive, wall facing pods. It does feel better, but too intimate for me. I don't want to face these two annoying, young, public-school boys who are far too confident, considering they've only just started working here. I want to get my head down and zone out in my own world.

I like working here. It's laid back. I came here for work experience and made myself so invaluable I never left. London's my back-up plan. If it doesn't work out here in Bristol, I'll go to where most of the documentary jobs are. For now, though, it's going pretty well. Each short contract in TV somehow leads on to another.

I like the city, too. It's small enough to feel like a village, and big enough to feel exciting. I mostly hang out in what the estate agents call the Golden Triangle: Clifton, Cotham, and Redland. The BBC, where I work, is on Whiteladies Road in Clifton. The buildings are mostly large, Georgian terraces with huge bay windows and tall ceilings. Bristol is built on a tidal estuary. The docks, once known for its trading of slaves, are now the cultural hub of the city. Old warehouses are now galleries, bars, cafés, and restaurants.

As a team, we don't really gel, unlike with the other two series I've worked on. There's no camaraderie. No in-jokes. Maybe that's why we were asked to move the desks around. I think it's because, secretly, we all think the series is crap and would rather be working on something better. It's not even for TV. It's a series of videos for a book publisher to profit from. I didn't get into this industry to help people make money. I want to be out on location filming important stories that change the world, not putting together this studio crap from the archive.

They're hungry for it, I'll give them that, the new boys. They've been given the opportunity to prove themselves. They're filling in temporarily because the director's been given the sack. She wasn't cutting it. I didn't think she was so bad; I liked her red hair and London style. I thought she was cool. But she's gone, and these two young upstarts, with practically no experience, have been given one of *my* programmes to rescue. Ironically the one called *Survival*. 'Survival' is too wide a subject to narrow down into an hour's storyline. We were struggling with it, the redhead and I. Coming up with a symbol, an animal or something that can represent the idea of survival was a challenge. Now these two wannabes are picking *my* brains for ideas. The fucking cheek. Get your own ideas! What's the point of taking the show away from me if you poach all my ideas?

I tell them my best one about using a survival kit as the main character. It could be animated, and the objects in it given human-like qualities: a pair of scissors walking across the screen, or a compass with its spinning point as a nose sniffing out the right direction. But they prefer the first off-the-top-of-my-head idea I had: a tortoise as the main character. A *tortoise?* How bloody obvious is that?

I can't wait to go to Ella's and get stoned. To tell her about these irritating researchers who think 'research' is 'asking other people for ideas'. She'll understand. She's on the same wavelength. We'll have a laugh, and a bitch, and I'll feel better about it.

Ella Richards works in TV as well. We met on the first researcher job I got here at the Beeb. She's tall and struts around in long leather boots looking like a brown haired Uma Thurman. She comes across as a bit snooty but I think it's just a defence mechanism. She's actually quite fun when you get to know her and she's cool. We had to make twenty short films for the BBC World Service, out of the most recent *Wildlife On One*s and *Natural World*s that had been released into the archive. For the first couple of years most programmes are embargoed but as soon as they've reached a certain age, all the footage becomes fair game. A bright spark in the Natural History Unit library set up this department to rehash old footage into new shows, which are then sold worldwide. The rest of the NHU look down on us folks here in Wildvision, but it's my training ground—I don't have a media studies degree.

I've been hanging out a lot with Ella ever since then, watching *Friends* on Friday nights, and talking about boys. She's just got together with Jake, a friend of Sol's. In fact, that's how I met Sol, through Ella. I think that's where she gets her weed from.

My neck's killing me. Coincidentally, an email pings round offering staff a ten-minute shiatsu massage. I don't know what that is, but as it's free I book myself in. I'm not officially staff, I'm just on a fixed term contract, but I figure that if I received the email, the offer must include me. In the meantime, an occupational therapist has arrived and is going round the room checking everyone's desks. When she gets to mine I tell her about my bad neck.

'There's a sharp pain when I turn my head,' I explain, turning it to the right.

'I'm not surprised,' she says. 'How long have you had your monitor at an angle like that?' I'm impressed. This woman's good; she's really sure of herself and makes it seem so obvious, I wonder why I hadn't realised myself. My monitor is to my left, in the corner of my desk, so it's not blocking off the two new guys sitting opposite. The keyboard is straight in front of me so I have to turn my head as I type, straining my right side.

'We all had to move our desks around last week,' I answer. The occupational therapist spends some time with me, making adjustments to my workspace. She talks about the importance of everything being angled and levelled so that our joints are at ninety degrees, allowing the circulation to flow smoothly. She moves my monitor so I don't need to turn my head, and lowers it so I don't have to look up. It's not rocket science but I thank her enthusiastically, grateful that the BBC provides this kind of support.

The shiatsu practitioner is not employed by the Beeb. He's come in to try his chances at finding new clients. I have no intention of becoming one, I just want the free treatment. He's Japanese. I'm not sure what I was expecting; I'm totally clueless about shiatsu. There's a special chair that I'm told to sit on. I have to straddle it and put my front up against the back of it—it's more comfortable than it looks. Without saying a word, he starts pummelling my shoulders as soon as I sit down. His hands feel very soft and skilled. He's so calm, I feel my thoughts racing in contrast. *Have I got time for this? I need to get back to work. What if he asks me to book a treatment? No, please don't pressure me to book a treatment! I'm not into this woo woo stuff. I've just got a bad neck from a badly positioned monitor. It's all explicable. There's nothing really wrong with me.*

My thoughts race on for the full ten minutes.

When the time is up he stands to the side with his hands clasped together. I get out of the chair and say, 'Thanks.' My shoulders feel totally different. I had no idea how much tension I was holding in them. He's not just fixed my neck, he's removed years of debris and lifted a weight I didn't even know I was carrying. I'm amazed. He doesn't give me any pushy sales crap either. He just smiles at me and does a little bow as if I am the most important person in his world right now. I didn't even catch his name.

* * *

My new director, Joe, arrived today. He's come from *Top Gear*. He's worked here before and all the old timers seem to know him. I can tell he's pleased to be back in the fold. He seems nice and his fiancée is called Emma, same as me. They're getting married very soon, he tells me, and she's been watching lots of movies where the woman is jilted at the altar. He feels exactly the same anxiety, worried that she'll be the one not to show up. Sweet couple, sharing their vulnerability with each other. I haven't really got a clue about relationships. I tell him about the liability I've been sleeping with. He's a musician with a band, record contract, album, and everything. I fall for that shit. A man who can play an instrument. He plays the double bass.

I remember a play by Patrick Süskind called *The Double Bass*, about a guy who treats his double bass like a girlfriend. Mainly because he's too shy to get a real one. Solomon's not like that. He's just a bit fucked up over his ex-girlfriend, Ruby, I tell Joe. His precious Ruby.

'Ruby?' Joe asks. 'Ruby Toogood?'

'Yes! Ruby Toogood! Do you know her?'

'We went to college together. They've been together for a long time. Ten years, I think.' Joe looks at me and seems to sense all that I'm hiding. The way I compare myself to Ruby even though I've never even met her. How I never feel good enough.

I met Sol this summer and he gave me one of those hand swipes only a black guy can get away with. He's actually white, so I thought it made him seem like he was trying too hard to be cool. We all piled down to East Prawle in Devon for a camping trip one weekend. We were off our heads, of course, and partying all night. When I went over to chat to him I could tell he fancied me. He seemed a little unsure of himself and it was quite endearing. It wasn't long before we were lying on the ground, his arm under my neck. It felt good, like all these severed connections between my head and my body rejoined.

A little later, a girl called Zanna with long dreadlocks and bright blue eyes arrived in a campervan. I don't know what gave it away, but I could tell she fancied Sol, too. I think it was in the way she was sizing me up, like I was her competition.

I'm not sure how much Sol and I have in common beyond the party scene. He went off to play a gig up north and didn't contact me when he got back, and I was hurt and confused. He said he thought I wasn't that into him. Maybe he was right—maybe I just wanted to be wanted. Anyway, I wouldn't let it go, I'm like a dog with a bone sometimes. I kept calling round his recording studio, which was opposite the pool I swim at. He had invited me once but I don't think he expected me to show up so often. Eventually we arranged to watch a video at mine, and I ended up giving him a massage. When I told Ella what happened she said, 'Oh my God! You seduced Solomon!' I hadn't seen it like that but I guess she was right. Anyway, it got me the invite to the avocado dinner, so my persistence paid off.

'So they've split up have they?' Joe continues, filling the awkward silence.

'Yeah. But he's not really over her,' I say, unable to hide my pain. I suddenly feel embarrassed. *He's* about to get married and *I'm* in a pathetic non-relationship with a man who's hung-up on his ex. I wish I'd kept my mouth shut. I'm such a gobshite! I don't want him to think I'm no good at my job because my personal life is a bit fucked up.

* * *

Joe's amazing! He's written a whole script and outline for the *Ocean* programme already. It's really visual and full of quirky effects to bring the sea alive onscreen. It shows how rubbish the redhead was. She didn't seem to do anything, come to think of it. Just looked a bit startled all the time. I felt sorry for her when they sacked her—it was a bit ruthless— but there's just no time to learn on the job. If you're the director, you're responsible for making the show. As a researcher I can get away with learning a little here and there, figuring out how to do the job by making it up as I go along. But if you can't write a script, and decide what to shoot and how to shoot it, then you haven't really got a programme.

It's my first hour-long documentary, and so far I've only been working on short films. I don't really know what I'm doing and I have this horrible feeling someone's going to find me out one day. I didn't go to Oxford or Cambridge like the rest of them; this place is full of public-school boys with corduroy elbow patches. I must stand out like a sore thumb with my northern accent. I don't even have a zoology degree—I went to Keele and read English and psychology. When I was deciding what degree to do, I thought zoology meant studying zoos. Everyone here's got a PhD in muntjac deer behaviour. I find all that a bit boring, so I don't really fit in.

I had absolutely no idea what the hell I was going to do when I finished uni. I had to ask myself a trick question to figure it out. 'What is it that I think only *other* people can do?' I asked myself. When I asked that question, I knew immediately. Documentary filmmaker. So I circled all the documentaries in the *TV Times* and watched them over a period of about three months. The ones I liked, I wrote down the name of the producer and production company from the credits, and sent them a letter. The story goes—and it may not be true because I might be remembering it wrong—I sent out 100 letters and I only got one reply. But that's all I needed, because it was from the BBC Natural History Unit in Bristol inviting me to do work experience.

I made myself invaluable during those three weeks. The series I was working on was going to be the first NHU programme to have a website, but the production team wasn't interested because computers were seen as 'techy' and for geeks. The woman who was building the site came to me in a fluster because the researchers on the show, who were supposed to provide her with content, had completely neglected to create any. The head of the BBC was coming especially to see this brand new all-singing, all-dancing website and all she had was the layout. So I got to work writing articles and making interactive games, which saved her bacon.

After that, she mentioned needing an assistant and told me to give my CV to her boss. I didn't bother because the internet wasn't a direction I wanted to go in. Then she showed up at my desk a week later saying she had pulled some strings to create the post especially for me and I couldn't get the job unless I actually applied. When I explained my reluctance she said that it was just a foot in the door, and she was absolutely right. I went on to get my first TV researcher job as a result; I also ended up moving in with her. I not only got a job, I got a flatmate to boot.

The truth is, I don't really want to make wildlife programmes. I'm more interested in people. But it's a great opportunity and I feel pretty cool telling people I work here as a researcher.

* * *

I hear everyone's going to the Mad Doc on Saturday so I go along, too. Nobody's invited me but I don't let that stop me. Sol is there and he kisses me on the cheek in a strange way when I arrive. I pick up something in the way he makes sure we don't kiss on the mouth in public and my stomach flips. Why did he do that? I know we're not officially an item, but there's no need to make a point of it!

He avoids me all evening, apart from one word he says to me as he's walking past on the dance floor. I think he's had quite a lot of coke. He has that arrogant swagger about him, all puffed up in his puffa jacket.

'Walkabout,' he says. That was it. Just walkabout. Like the Aborigines do. It sounded passive-aggressive. He might have meant he'd been for a walkabout or was going on walkabout but he said it more like a command. *Walkabout.* Keep your eyes open and figure out what's happening here. I'm too fucked up to be honest with you to tell you. You'll have to find out for yourself.

It's funny, how I find out. We're all in a taxi going home: me, Sol, Zanna, and Nat. Zanna gets out first. She looks surprised and confused that no one else is getting out of the cab with her, but she doesn't say anything. When I get out, a little further on, Sol stays in the taxi with Nat, and it's my turn to look confused. I don't want the night to end. I still want to party, so I walk round to Zanna's. I figure she'll be pleased to see me because she looked like she wasn't expecting the night to be over either. She is pleased. We get a fire going, and chat about the night not being over, wondering why the guys went home to bed, because it wasn't like them.

'Sol was weird tonight,' I say. 'Was Ruby there?' I haven't met Ruby so I don't know what she looks like. Her being at the club would explain why Sol greeted me strangely. Maybe he didn't want his ex-girlfriend to see us together.

'Are *you* sleeping with him, too?' Zanna asks gently. The penny drops. My stomach squeezes tight around the shock and I suddenly feel stupid and angry. I'd seen them together during the evening, Zanna leaning on Sol's back as he was crouched down talking to Nat, but I brushed it aside as just a friendship. I must have known unconsciously what was going on. That's why I was at her flat, to find out. So here we are, rivals, in the same boat, caught in the wake of Solomon's inability to communicate.

A few days later, I go round to Solomon's to score some weed. An old friend from uni wants me to get him a bag of skunk and Solomon grows the stuff. It's a good excuse to go round and see what's what. I haven't seen him since the taxi home. I get another shock as I walk through the door because Zanna is there. I pretend I'm cool, but I'm hurt, and the vibe I get from Sol, loud and clear, is *don't come around to my flat uninvited, because you might not like what you see.* He doesn't say it in words but I can sense it in him. And Zanna is acting like I'm not even there.

Nat invites me in and offers me a game of chess. I don't know why I do it to myself but I sit down and help lay out the chess pieces.

'Are you OK?' Nat asks considerately, passing me a spliff.

'Yeah,' I say, lying. Solomon and Zanna are lying on the bed, all playful together, with their feet touching sole to sole and giggling as if they're alone. The dope bends my head and I can't concentrate. The game doesn't last long. Nat castles his king with an elaborate gesture that seems totally fitting. Sol the king in his castle with Zanna his new queen, and Nat closing in on me, the pawn.

Next move, I'm in checkmate.

'Check mate.'

No mates here.

I take the bag of weed and head home. I look at the silvery green leaves and think, fuck it, I'm going to smoke the whole bag! And when I'm finished, I'm going to quit once and for all.

CHAPTER TWO

Insomnia

It's 3am and I can't sleep. Time has become nothing more than a measure of how many hours' sleep I will get if I fall asleep right now. My mind, like the clock, does not stop ticking. I don't know where the off switch is in my head. Looking for it is the very opposite of finding it. The only thing that is going to do the trick is a spliff, but I'm not succumbing. I knew insomnia would grip me, my brain reclaiming its freedom after seven years of being in a cannabis fog. I've tried to give it up a few times but it's always the same. The sleeplessness kicks in and I usually give in. Not this time! I'm determined to see this through, whatever the outcome.

I turn over to find a new position, a fresh attempt at getting to sleep. But I know it's useless. I don't know how to relax. Irrelevant sentences are chugging around my head, filling the void of night-time nothingness.

The time pressures of deadlines, the *need-it-done-yesterday* attitude of working in TV, not feeling good enough, always feeling fearful that I'm going to be found out, have put my nervous system on red alert. I feel like I'm playing a constant video game. Quick responses, instant decisions, no time to hesitate, no time to wait, and rest, and let the wisdom in.

My thoughts are whirring away like a ceiling fan on the highest setting. Time passes but I remain stuck in the stretched out night of an insomniac. I will be like this in an hour; I was like this an hour ago. Sleep can't find me, and I can't find sleep.

Anger sets in after hours of predictable boredom. I'm angry with sleep, angry about insomnia, and angry with myself. Four hours to go before I have to get up for work. I've no chance now and that means I will be a mess tomorrow. Having to get up in the morning is adding a tension to the situation that I decide to remove. If I don't get any sleep, I'll call in sick.

Letting myself off the hook doesn't bring the oblivion I crave. By 8am I'm still wide awake. I'm relieved the night is over, though. At least I can get out of this waiting room and face the day.

* * *

I hear through the grapevine that Sol has broken his leg. *It serves him right*, I think. Without making any arrangements, I head to the hospital and am told to wait in a room along the corridor from his ward. There are a few kids' toys strewn around the floor. Two women are there with their toddlers. A gorgeous little girl with blonde curls and big blue eyes, who can't be more than three years old, approaches me.

'You're all sea horsey,' she says.

'What does she mean?' I ask her mother.

'I've no idea.' She's picking up on something that I haven't recognised in myself. I definitely feel *kind of sea horsey*, a bit wobbly and out at sea.

Solomon's bed is surrounded by a big gang of his friends, including Zanna and Nat. I'm not sure if I'm welcome but they all act pleased to see me anyway. Some situations allow water to pass quickly under the bridge and this feels like one of them.

'What happened?' I ask, and Sol launches into some great skateboarding tale. I look at him blankly, not understanding any of the street jargon. I'm not as impressed by it as he was hoping. I think he's perhaps too old for skating around like a teenager. I can tell he's exaggerating the danger so his leg break is more justifiable.

'What would you say if I told you that I went to school with that guy over there?' Sol points to the man in the bed opposite him. Solomon was brought up in Bristol so I don't think it's such a big deal that he knows someone on his ward, but he's obviously surprised by it. The man is in all kinds of contraptions with a button in his hand, which he clicks to get another shot of morphine. Everyone is looking at me for my response, as if they're expecting me to have the definitive answer.

'Well, if I was insane,' I say sarcastically, 'I'd think Mystic Meg had just won the lottery!' My brain is working so quickly, I barely understand my own joke but everybody laughs even though it doesn't quite make sense.

* * *

It's the NHU Christmas ball and I don't want to miss it. For someone who hasn't slept for three nights, I don't feel very tired. I put on a bright green dress that I bought off my flatmate. I don't know why she didn't like it. Something about the colour she said. It didn't suit her. I think it's because it's so short. I decide not to wear any underwear just to balance out the feeling of formality of the occasion. It's not like me, but the insomnia is taking its toll. I put on some black nylon tights and high heel shoes and get a taxi to the posh hotel venue.

My friend Kate is there, looking stunning in a crimson red satin dress. She tells me about the couple of grand she just won on a lottery ticket and her subsequent shopping spree, hence the outfit. Kate is another tall BBC colleague who towers above me. She has cropped, pixie-like dark hair and sparkly eyes that turn up at the corners when she smiles. She used to go out with Jake, who Ella is now going out with. Apparently he came on really strong to Ella and she said he was hard to resist. It's good to see Kate looking so gorgeous now though; it must have been hard for her. They were together for a long time. *Ten years* I think, *like Sol and Ruby.*

The party is pretty boring otherwise, and I feel awkward and out of place, so I leave early and go round to Ella's. She said I could stay the night with her if I couldn't sleep at mine. She rents a top floor flat in Clifton, the swankiest part of town. It's tiny and the windows are only half-sized, sash ones, made especially small to fit an attic, but I love that she's got her own place. It seems so grown-up to live on your own.

I share her double bed and wrap my feet around hers, like sea horses do. But it's useless. I can't sleep there either.

I've no idea what time it is. I get up to go to the loo but Jake is sitting on the toilet with the lid down. It's not actually him, not in the flesh, but some kind of ghost of him. He looks like he's made of purply green light, not totally solid, but not see-through either. He's just sitting there using the toilet as a seat, waiting for me. He says something that doesn't really make sense but makes perfect sense to *me*. He says, in a deep, gurgling, kind of way,

'Do not disturb undisturbed men.'

I think he's referring to Sol. He means I should not have disturbed Sol because he wasn't ready to be disturbed. He's basically telling me not to knock on men's doors for a relationship when they're not ready for one. It's good advice and makes a lot of sense. I'm not in the least bit fazed that I've seen some kind of strange apparition—but I don't tell anyone about it either.

In the morning, Ella takes me to the GP for some sleeping tablets. I need her to do the talking. The doctor says not to worry, I probably am sleeping, I just don't realise it. *How does he know?* He prescribes tranquillisers, even though I need sleeping tablets, but I can't speak and I just skip out of his office winking like a pixie.

Back at my flat I look at the bottle of pills. Take as directed the label says. How the fuck was I directed? My head's fried. I take one and hope for the best.

They don't work. Still no sleep.

* * *

I started smoking dope at uni. It gave me a sense of community. Moving around so often as a child, I felt like I didn't really belong anywhere.

I was born in India and after six months we moved to Nigeria for three years and then the Ivory Coast for another three, so I didn't actually live in England until I was nearly seven. Dad worked for what used to be ICI—Imperial Chemical Industries—selling dye, mostly indigo from India, for denim. With the rise in fashion for jeans, there was a global market to tap. He enjoyed travelling the world in a way that allowed him to take his family along and still be well provided for. So we were expats, foreigners overseas but no longer fitting into our own country, either.

When I was thirteen, we moved again, this time to Hong Kong. It was a British colony, fought-for in the nineteenth century as a port for the British Empire to trade opium from India to China. Drugs were rife there in the Eighties. In 1983, when we arrived, there were government information ads on TV showing what your son or daughter might look like if they were heroin addicts. They put me off; back then, I was totally against drugs.

At sixteen, my best friend announced she was going off to boarding school for the sixth form. It was a tradition in her family, to prepare the kids for university, so I decided I wanted to go to boarding school as well. I convinced my parents, and myself, that it was because Dad had only signed another year's contract and I didn't want to risk having to go back to the UK, thus changing schools and syllabuses, halfway though my A Levels. But the truth was, I couldn't picture myself in the sixth form without her.

It wasn't until I went to Keele that I gravitated towards dope smoking. Being stoned helped me stop worrying about what I ate. I'd been dieting for years and was obsessed by what I was or wasn't allowed to consume. Getting the munchies and stuffing our faces with chocolate bars, biscuits, and toast in the early hours of the morning was not only fun, it actually sorted out what could have otherwise turned into a more serious eating disorder. I saw breaking free from my over-controlling ways as a positive step. I was challenging the oversimplified story I'd been given, that drugs were bad for you.

But now the drugs might just be my downfall. Well, giving them up, at least.

I call my old friend from uni, Claire, who's practical, level-headed, and above all non-judgmental. She has a laugh that sings in her throat and an honesty that makes her safe. She's a straight-talking northerner who tells it like it is. I need to speak to her about the invite to her fiancé's surprise birthday party this coming weekend. With the insomnia, I don't think I'll be able to make it.

I don't remember mentioning death to Claire on the phone. But alone in my room, afterwards, I definitely think about it. I think about the book I read in the final year of my psychology degree called *Why We Sleep*. It said that no one had ever died through lack of sleep but they had gone a little crazy, paranoid. I'm not afraid of that. But I am afraid of death.

I haven't slept for four nights now. Maybe I'll be the first person to die from not sleeping. I can't imagine not existing. It's not in my ability to because the thing that imagines it would have to not be there. I lie down on my bed, overwhelmed by the physics.

Head fuck.

My head is all over the place and I keep checking the curtains, imagining I'm seeing Ella waiting in her car at the junction across the road. But why would she be spying on me? Is it her way of looking out for me?

When I call Claire to tell her I won't make it to the party, mentioning death rings alarm bells and she sends her fiancé, Chris, down to see how I am. But she doesn't tell me he's coming.

I'm lying on my bed thinking about Sol. To help me get to sleep, Ella has told me to think of the person I want to spend the rest of my life with and wait right there, and the only person I can think of to think of is Sol. There's a knock at the door. *Sol?* I think, kicking off the covers and tentatively making my way to the door.

It's Chris, with his spectacles perched on the end of his long nose.

He's not the person I'm supposed to spend the rest of my life with! I look at him sheepishly. He's going to marry Claire!

'What are *you* doing here, Chris? You'll miss your surprise party!' I blurt out, ruining the surprise. Oops.

I invite him in and, thinking his psychology degree gives him some kind of insight into human behaviour, I chew his ear off about all that's happened. I tell him all the minute details, hoping he'll be able to figure out how Solomon feels about me. But Chris doesn't have any answers. He just listens.

I graduated the year before Chris but met him the following year when he was doing his finals. Some friends from that year had set up a radio station at the university, so I went to help them out. I crashed on Chris's sofa and noticed lots of people coming and going for computer help. Chris was a whiz-kid who had written some computer program when he was fourteen. Nobody had their own computers, and email had only just arrived on the scene. He spent so much time helping other people with word processing for their dissertations, he neglected his own. Because I'd also done psychology, I helped out with the experiments he didn't manage to show up for. Claire, who was only his girlfriend back then, was away in Australia travelling. She was the rock in their relationship and without her he struggled to take care of himself. Claire had been grateful for the support I gave Chris while she was away. Without my help, he might not have completed his psychology dissertation.

Now it's my turn to need help, and Kate and Chris are doing what good friends do: taking the initiative to support me in my hour of need.

Once I've finished babbling on about Sol, Chris and I sit in silence on the sofa. Suddenly, a strange scene plays out in my mind's eye, like an overlay onto the room. It's not a hallucination because I'm seeing it inside my head. But it's not *exactly* an image I'm seeing. It's more a feeling of a long-forgotten memory, a snapshot from another lifetime. It *feels* like I'm sitting in a circle with the people I know in Bristol. They're not the same people as they are now because I get the impression we're in a different century. Yet somehow I *know* they're the same people. They send me out to run sexual errands for them. In return they look after me, giving me shelter, clothing, and food, a practical arrangement for our mutual survival. For a nanosecond I feel a sinister abusive entanglement with my Bristol friends that I can't quite pinpoint, but it has something to do with this odd flashback.

The image fades and the room returns to normal.

What the fuck was all that about? It must be the lack of sleep. I go to my room telling Chris I'm going to bed because it's late, though sleep still doesn't feel possible. I pace around nervously then stop in the middle of my room, quivering. I'm shaking like a leaf.

* * *

Friday the thirteenth. Still no sleep. Chris seems keen to find my flat-mate for reasons that don't get explained and I don't think to ask. We get into his car and he asks me where she's likely to be.

'She's probably at her boyfriend's flat, not far from here.' Chris asks for directions and starts the engine. Driving around Cotham, I pretend not to remember where her boyfriend lives. I don't want to see him. He laughed at the state of me when he was round at our place the other day. I think it was just out of embarrassment but still it was most *un*helpful. I purposely take Chris on a wild goose chase. I look down a street as if vaguely remembering it so that he'll drive down that way. It works. He turns down the wrong street. After doing this a few times, he gets frustrated and I'm secretly revelling in his struggle. Serves him right for not communicating with me! But I don't know how I'm going to keep this up. I need to get away from this stupid situation.

I grab the handle of the car door and make a quick run for it. Chris soon comes speeding after me looking really frustrated, like he's looking after a child that won't do as it's told. Realising I can't get away that easily, I get back into the car and Chris drives us back to my flat.

He marches into my bedroom asking what clothes I want to pack and reaches for a jumper on the shelf. He's probably just scared, but to me he looks pissed off. I don't know what we're packing for so I'm not very helpful. He stuffs some clothes and underwear into a bag and then we're getting in his car again.

It's a cold, bleak winter's day and the atmosphere inside the car is just as icy.

We're heading up north, presumably, to my parents' house. They live on the edge of Manchester, in a small village, almost in the Peak District. It couldn't be more different from the chaos that is my Bristol life.

Chris calls Claire and has a strained conversation with her.

'We're on our way back,' he says, tensely. I know he wants to tell her what a nightmare he's having but he says he's fine.

'See you soon,' he says, hanging up.

My hands feel cold, especially my forefinger, like a dead man's finger. I rub it to warm it up but I feel like I'm giving Chris a secret sign that I'm pulling his plonker, so I stop. The seat warms up beneath me and I'm not sure if it's perhaps me.

'What's happening with the seat?'

'It's heated.'

'It feels weird. Like I've wet myself.'

'Yeah. It is a bit strange if you're not used to it. Do you want me to switch it off?'

'No. It's good. I'm cold.'

We stop at a service station.

'Air and water,' I say. Chris takes it as a command to check the air and water but I'm half saying it to myself, reminding myself of my basic needs.

We walk into the hyper-real hyper-fake foyer. Christmas decorations and novelty tunes carry me into a world of jolly shoppers but I have no interest in buying anything. Chris buys me a Coke and sits down at a table. I join him and he looks relieved. I glug the drink down through the straw.

'Coke, I love Coke.' I slurp the last drops noisily through the ice cubes realising I've no idea if I've eaten or drunk anything since the insomnia began. 'I'm just going off to wait for a signal,' I say. I see Chris visibly give up trying to control me and then I head for the door where a big padded Santa is jiggling a bucket. Claire! Chris's fiancée! She's smiling at me through this Santa disguise. I know it's not her dressed as Santa but somehow she's managing to smile *through* his eyes. Santa shakes the bucket of coins and nods at me. That's the signal. Claire is leading us home. All is well. I head back to where Chris is sitting and we make a move to leave.

When we get to my parents' house, it's late. I barely notice the familiar stone walls of the house I grew up in, exposed now the leaves of the Virginia creeper have dropped off for the winter. I have no words to explain what's happening to me so I flop down at the doorway closing my eyes. Mum rushes to my side, concern creasing her forehead. She looks older than her fifty-one years, her grey hairs hiding under the brown hair dye—not that I notice this right now. I'm somewhere else in a delusional reality. I think that perhaps I'm a drug addict here to get some heroin from the surgery where Mum works on reception.

Dad is here too, commanding without having a clue what to do in the situation. He's normally the one in charge: logical, practical, and confident. But it's my sister, Sally, who leads on this rare occasion. She's never been that self-assured, usually looking to the outside world for affirmation. She's there with her husband and I'm not sure if they just happen to be there or have heard I'm on my way and want to help. They're all crowding around me, discussing what to do. There is some talk about the tablets I'm taking and how many I've had. I've given them to Chris to look after and he must have handed them over. The bottle is full as I only took one last night. Surely they'll be able to work that out. I haven't overdosed. Do they think I've overdosed?

Sally seems the most sure about what to do. I'm impressed with her unusual assertiveness. It's probably her emergency training as cabin crew.

'We need to call an ambulance, and get her to hospital—she could have overdosed,' she pronounces authoritatively.

Jesus Christ! I'm not suicidal! But I can't speak.

'Pixie me,' I say to Mum, winking. 'Pixie me, pixie me,' is the most sense I can muster but even I know it doesn't make sense.

Sally dials a number, and waits.

* * *

Mum sits with me in the ambulance with a worried look on her face. Mental and emotional health is outside her range of expertise. She trained as a nurse before she had children, but gave it up halfway through, to have my elder brother, Solomon (there is more than one Solomon in my life). She knows about physical ailments and whenever we were sick, as kids, she always knew what to do. She actually had dreams of being a midwife and went back to do her nursing training again once we were all happily settled at school. But she gave it up a second time, halfway through, when we moved to Hong Kong.

Mum knows the NHS and ambulances and hospitals. But now, she makes pointless conversation with the ambulance men and they act all chipper and jolly. I hate the way she's being so fake with them. I feel angry with her for being so nice when I can see she's worried sick. The incongruence is confusing. She keeps flicking her eyes over my way and back to them.

Maybe she's worried about the ambulance men.

Maybe they're abducting us. Maybe they're going to rape us!

* * *

The junior doctor can't get any sense out of me when he asks me if I know who I am. He leads us to a separate waiting room, an almost-bare space with two chairs and a cheap Formica table. It's not private, but it's clear to me that there won't be anyone else allowed in while we're in there. He tells us to wait for Ravi Shankar, the psychiatrist on duty.

Ravi Shankar? Who plays sitar with The Beatles?

I pace around the box-like room feeling anxious. It's stark and bright. Scribblings appear on the walls, sentences covering every bit of space. I can't read the words because the faded biro letters are too small. It looks like different people have added to it over the years. A wall of solidarity, graffiti from all those who have waited here before. I know I'm the only one who can see these messages but, ironically, they tell me I'm not alone. For a moment I'm reassured but my eyes dart to a bomb alert poster on the door. A bomb alert? The warning sends my body into a panic. My bladder quivers and I feel a sudden gush downwards. I stand in the middle of the room as warm liquid trickles down through my clothes and onto the vinyl floor.

Mum herds me off to a nearby toilet to clean up the mess. I've started my period, too. I form a strange repeating gesture with my hands, trying to show eggs coming out of my ovaries and down my fallopian tubes. I've no idea what I'm doing and Mum has no way of understanding either.

'How do you know I'm not Ella Richards?' I ask her, still repeating the hand gesture.

'I know you're not Ella Richards,' Mum answers.

'But *how* do you know?'

'I know who you are. You're not Ella Richards,' she says, frustrated. She leaves me in the bathroom for a short while whilst she goes off to find me something dry to put on.

Once I'm changed, Ravi Shankar, the psychiatrist, arrives. It's not *the* Ravi Shankar. I'm thrown because I thought Ravi was a man's name. I wasn't expecting a woman.

She asks me three questions. I've heard about these questions. A friend of my mum's told my mum about them when her son went mad from cannabis. Mum never told me what they were, just that her friend had been really impressed because it enabled them to ascertain whether you're sane or not.

The first question.

'Do you know who you are?' I enjoy the existential conundrum but find no answer small enough to put into words. I beam at the psychiatrist, shrugging my shoulders.

She asks me the second question.

'Do you know how you got here?' I've no idea how any of us got here. Big Bang? Evolution? I shrug again.

The third and final question.

'Do you know who I am?' Her tone emphasises the gravity of the situation.

Is she really Ravi Shankar? Are they playing a trick on me? She's not *the* Ravi Shankar but she's wearing a name badge so I best go along with it. I nod and smile as if to say hey, I'm in on the joke.

I'm admitted to ward P2 at 2am on Saturday, December 14, 1996, after the strangest Friday the 13th ever.

CHAPTER THREE

Admission

The air brushes gently against my cheeks as I'm wheeled down an interminably long corridor, even though I can walk, to ward P2. P stands for 'Psychiatric'. I'm taken to a small room that has a single bed, a sink, a chest of drawers, and a notice board. I ask Mum to pin up my wet, bloodstained knickers on the board as I get into bed.

A different doctor arrives. I'm given an injection. That does it. I'm fading now, losing my grip. The air in the room is thick and white, like I'm seeing through dry ice. The Indian doctor and my dad are moving around and talking over me. I can't make out what they're saying. I experience a weird flashback that I'm in Breach Candy Hospital, Bombay, where I was born. Perhaps I'm going to be reborn.

My mind is slipping away into the distance. After five nights, I'm finally asleep.

* * *

I wake in the middle of the night to find that I've wet the bed. I used to wet the bed when I was a kid, until I was eleven. Eventually the GP gave me some tranquillisers to take before I went to sleep. When I asked Mum what they were she said they were something that would have the opposite effect when I was an adult. So this is what she meant. They make you pee the bed!

I wrap myself up in the wet sheet, holding all four edges so that I'm completely hidden inside, like I'm in a bag. I slip out through the door and into the corridor. Crawling along the edge, where the wall meets the floor, I make sure I remain covered so that the wet patch is clearly visible. It's a deliberate act of self-humiliation, exposing the messy evidence for all to see.

A nurse comes over and finds her way into the sheet.

'What are you doing in there, love?' She ushers me back into my room and then goes off to get clean bedding and returns with an efficiency that tells me it's all part of a night's work.

Alone again, I sit up in bed. Like a three year old at fantasy play, I go along with the urge to act out a strange game of charades. I grab the top right hand corner of the sheet and make a shape that I cradle in one arm—a baby. I don't really know what I'm doing or why. Improvisation is just happening and it's easiest to go along with it. I grab the opposite top left hand corner and make another shape and cup it in my other arm—another baby. Twins. It doesn't make sense but the charade seems to be over even though I haven't figured it out yet.

I get out of bed, quietly open my bedroom door again, and poke my head out, careful not to attract any attention. At the end of the corridor I see two cots. After scrutinising, I see that they're actually laundry baskets but in this game they're representing cots. Twins again. But these twins are the ones my mother had in her first pregnancy. Born prematurely, these two girls died only a few hours after they were born. Why am I seeing them down the corridor? I bring my head back into the room and close the door gently. Maybe my psyche is trying to tell me something, but I've no idea what the hell it is.

I look into the mirror for reassurance. I peer into my reflection, smoothing my face with my hands. Leaning in closer, the skin on my forehead looks dry, aging me. I'm twenty-seven and starting to get wrinkles! I have exactly the same frown line as my mum, a knife wound in the centre of my brow, deep and sharp. How do genes do that, create exactly the same frown line? It looks like years of troubled thinking. I'm starting to look just like my mother.

'You *are* beautiful.' A voice from somewhere to the back of my head, it could have even been behind me. But there's no one else in the room. The most beautiful voice I've ever heard. She sounds angelic. It's definitely not just a thought in my head. It's audible, and would register in my auditory cortex but probably isn't perceptible to others. A voice only I can hear, like a guardian angel, taking care of me in my hour of need. And for a moment, I wonder if she's right. Maybe I am beautiful.

In the morning, I put what few clothes I have away in the drawers, making labels for them, 'under wearer bearer drawer', 'top shop'. I don't have many things. I don't think Chris packed for this.

A student psychiatrist comes to see me. She's wearing black. I don't like black right now. It makes me feel afraid.

'You are all in black,' I say. Quick as a flash, she opens up her cardigan revealing a bright red top.

'Oh, but I'm red underneath,' she replies.

Red is good. She has a warm heart.

* * *

There's an old lady sitting by my bed that I barely recognise. I know it's my mum, but it's like I'm seeing her for the first time, really looking at her properly. Her hands are deeply lined with the evidence of a lifelong schedule of housework. She's wearing glasses to read and is engrossed in her book so doesn't notice me looking at her. I don't exist to her in this state. I'm an imposter and she's waiting for her daughter to return.

She's brought me an advent calendar to help me keep track of the days. It has lights and music and looks magical. I circle December 13th. The day Chris drove me to my parents. The day I lost the plot. It is the last day I knew what day it was. I write 'definitely Groundhog Day' across the day's door and fold it open. I don't know how long I've been in hospital so I don't know how many other doors to open. I look around the room for clues. The *Telegraph* that Dad left behind is on the floor by my bed. That will have a date on it! But I don't know when he left it there. Was it yesterday or today? It could be an old paper, a few days old, even. It's no use. I'm only trying to race ahead. Race ahead into the future where I'm better. Racing my own head.

* * *

My brother Sol, his wife, and baby daughter have come to visit with Mum and Dad. They're up north for Christmas. They put my niece on the bed and nervously corral her so she doesn't fall off. They've brought me a present, a Winnie-the-Pooh pottery making set. It's for children aged six and up. I can see their thinking. It's something for me to do in hospital. Sol knows I'm into Winnie-the-Pooh but obviously doesn't realise that it's because I read *The Tao of Pooh* and that I'm more interested in Taoism than in Disney.

Sol looks awkward. He doesn't look at all like the Solomon I know. I've never seen him look so uncomfortable. His head moves like it's trying to avoid being there, like he wants to disappear but finding that impossible, his face contorts into both fear and friendliness, having a battle with itself.

'You're not Sol,' is all I can think of to say.

'I am Sol.' He wriggles, squirming with embarrassment.

'No, you're not.' I'm trying to say that he doesn't look like I've ever seen him look. These awkward gestures are entirely new movements that I've never seen him do before so he's not the Solomon I know. Everyone else is quiet. Maybe they think I was expecting to see the other Solomon, the one I've been sleeping with.

'I am Sol.'

'No you're not Sol.'

'I am.'

My brother and I used to argue a lot when we were kids. Neither of us could ever see eye to eye. In the end he usually said, 'You always have to get the last word in don't you?' It always shut me up because that meant he was wrong. I didn't need to get the last word in—he did!

Older now, I end the pointless to-ing and fro-ing that's getting us nowhere.

'If you are who you say you are, please leave now.' I'm trying to trick them into revealing Solomon isn't really being himself but everyone gets up without saying a word and walks out of the room.

Now I'm alone. The room feels deathly empty. That didn't go well.

* * *

I've been prescribed anti-psychotic medication. Something called Halo-peridol. I'm not sectioned so technically I have the right to refuse treatment, but that is just a technicality. When I do refuse, they find creative ways of making me take it.

'Open wide,' says the cheerful nurse who wheels his bike down the corridor every morning. I trust him and wonder what fun game we're playing. He squirts a disgusting liquid from a plastic syringe. It looks like urine and tastes bitter as hell and I feel tricked, my trust betrayed.

Injecting me in the bottom is less deceptive but requires more force. I don't like either method. Now, I go up to the drug counter and say, 'Hallo Peridol,' obediently opening my mouth. I swallow hard then lift my tongue to show that the pill's gone down. It's all a sarcastic show of compliance but I'd rather take it disgruntled than against my will.

It clamps the muscles in my back, pulls my arms in to my sides with bent elbows, and makes me shuffle. I look like a zombie puppet. I can tell who else is taking it by the way they shuffle too. The Haloperidol Shuffle. If we weren't mad when we arrived, we certainly look it now.

It's the main thing that distinguishes us from the staff. Nobody wears a uniform on this ward. It's meant to make it seem more relaxed. But it just confuses the visitors.

Dad and I play a game. Who's the patient and who's a member of staff? Can he tell the difference? It's easy for me. I know intuitively plus the staff don't usually hang out around the corridors. They're only ever there for a reason, to attend to something. The rest of the time they hide away in the office.

'He's a member of staff,' Dad says pointing to Dirty Pete.

'No way. He's a patient.'

'Are you sure?' Dad doesn't like being wrong.

'Absolutely. Just because he's wearing a waistcoat? Don't be fooled. He's definitely a patient. His name's Pete. I call him Dirty Pete because he gives me the creeps. It's him that blasts out that marching band music full volume.' Dirty Pete has intense, dark, grey semi-circles under his eyes. His skin has a grey hue to it. He came up to me on my first day and did a disturbing impression of me crawling down the corridor, breathing with horror movie-like exaggerated sound effects of me sliding along the floor.

'Please don't do that,' I said. 'It's hard enough being in this place without having to deal with you doing that.' He instantly transformed into a friendly bloke and insisted on taking me to see his old record player. He always plays the same tune, one that sounds like a circus intro. He likes to put it on full volume, announcing another day at the circus.

The ward is like a circus. There's the Fabulous Furry Freak Brother who sits on the same chair, all day every day. His long hair is a mess but hides his face. He doesn't look at anyone or talk to anyone. Just sits there smoking roll ups. Dancing Man glides along, with his hands splayed wide like jazz hands wearing, white gloves.

'Do you have a sister called Sally?' He asks me.

'Yes,' I reply, wondering how he knows her.

'She was in my class at school.'

'Right,' I say, wishing I were anonymous. I'm not exactly proud to be on this psych ward.

The Old Feather Lady lies on her bed being pumped full of oxygen so that when she gets up, she's so light she looks like she floats out of the room. She only gets up for a cigarette and then gets straight back into bed for more oxygen. There's Football Fan, who likes to wear his Man U T-shirt on his head, and there's Mavis. Mavis tells me she tried to hang herself in the bathroom using the light switch cord.

'That's a stupid way to try to kill yourself,' I reply unsympathetically. She obviously just wants attention or else why would she bother telling me? If she really wanted to top herself she'd find a more effective method. The most disturbing though is The Mad Woman In The Attic. She arrives one day and sits outside the meeting room and insists on being allowed to see the doctor immediately. The consultant only jets in once every couple of weeks so she has a long wait on her hands. For the entire day she sits there stubbornly refusing to budge.

'My husband brought me in here,' she yells. 'I'm not mad. I want to see the doctor NOW. My husband thinks I'm crazy but there's absolutely nothing wrong with me.' She's still there the next day. I can't decide whether she's crazy or her husband is a controlling bastard who can't deal with her emotions. It's disturbing to witness. She's fucked either way, isn't she? If there's nothing wrong with her then her husband has powers he shouldn't have. Or if she's no idea she's doolally, then how's she ever going to get herself better?

What we all share, despite our differences, is being on the receiving end of the total failure on the part of the mental health service to help us to deal with the distress we are in. On the contrary, our very distress is pathologised as if there is something inherently wrong with us. We are viewed as a collection of diagnoses, derogatory labels, a 'them' distinct from the 'us' that must be medicated back to normality. If you don't want to take medication you're 'non-compliant' and seen as a nuisance, a menace even. There must be something wrong with you if you deny your need for medication. Your denial is very proof of your insanity and delusional state.

Something has flipped inside me—but not in the way that they think. There's a horrible moment when I see in their eyes how I'm being perceived, like realising you're facing a dictator who you have to go along with in order not to be shot. Taking the medication is hard enough, but not taking it is even harder. In fact it's not possible, once you're in the clutches of the psychiatric system. There is no other option. It's all they know, and all they've been taught. In any other department in the hospital it would be explained to you what they're going to give you, why, the effect it's going to have, and any possible side effects. Here, on this ward, I've lost that privilege.

* * *

There's a famous experiment called the Rosenhan experiment, named after the psychologist David Rosenhan, the Stanford University professor who conducted it. It was published by the journal *Science* in 1973 under the title 'On being sane in insane places'. He wanted to determine the validity of psychiatric diagnosis. The study was done in two parts. The first part involved the use of healthy 'pseudopatients' (three women and five men, including Rosenhan himself) who briefly feigned auditory hallucinations in an attempt to gain admission to twelve different psychiatric hospitals in five different states in various locations in the United States. All were admitted and diagnosed with psychiatric disorders. After admission, the pseudopatients acted normally and told staff that they felt fine and had no longer experienced any additional hallucinations. All were forced to admit to having a mental illness, and forced to agree to take antipsychotic drugs as a condition of their release.

During their initial psychiatric assessment, the pseudopatients claimed to be hearing voices of the same sex as the patient, which were often unclear, but which seemed to pronounce the words 'empty', 'hollow', 'thud', and nothing else. These words were chosen as they vaguely suggested some sort of existential crisis, and for the lack of any published literature referencing them as psychotic symptoms. No other psychiatric symptoms were claimed. Despite constantly and openly taking extensive notes on the behaviour of the staff and other patients, none of the pseudopatients were identified as impostors by the hospital staff, although many of the other psychiatric patients seemed to be able to correctly identify them as impostors. Hospital notes indicated that staff interpreted much of the pseudopatients' behaviour in terms of mental illness. For example, one nurse labelled the note-taking as 'writing behaviour' and considered it pathological.

Rosenhan and the other pseudopatients reported an overwhelming sense of dehumanisation, severe invasion of privacy, and boredom while hospitalised. They reported that though the staff seemed to be well-meaning, they often discussed them at length in their presence as though they were not there, and avoided direct interaction except as strictly necessary to perform official duties.

This is exactly how I was treated in 1996, twenty-three years after this study was published.

The second part of the research involved a hospital administration that was offended by the claims, and challenged Rosenhan to send pseudopatients to its facility, which its staff would then detect. Rosenhan agreed and, in the following weeks, out of 193 new patients, the staff identified forty-one as potential pseudopatients. In fact, Rosenhan had sent no pseudopatients to the hospital.

The study concluded, 'It is clear that we cannot distinguish the sane from the insane in psychiatric hospitals,' and also illustrated the dangers of dehumanisation and labelling in psychiatric institutions.

* * *

I wake early in the morning with the sounds of the night shift change over. It's still dark outside, the curtains blocking out the glare from the orange street light. There's a faint purple glow around the drapes. An aura. I stare at it looking for its source. It's not the moon. There's a midnight blueness to the light, the kind of blue that lighting departments might use to create the effect of night-time on a film set. There's also purple—a royal purple, almost indigo, around the edges of the nylon fabric. I thought only living things had auras. Man-made fibres don't have auras, do they?

Later, my family visits again. They come every day with pale pink tulips and get-well cards from friends in Bristol. My wall is covered with well wishes, colourful images, and a lot of love. Mum has brought me a DVD to watch. We go into one of the lounges, a quiet one that's on the geriatric wing because no one else is in there. I lie down on the floor, my head resting in my hands and I lose myself in the rhythms and tappings of *Riverdance*. The loud drums and short, sharp fiddle beat the time for the perfectly straight-backed women with loose legs that crisscross and flick out the Irish jig.

The others get a bit bored and chat among themselves. The music is very dramatic and I am mesmerised because I see them again. All the dancers have auras, beautiful purple halos around their bodies. I don't say anything because it's obvious no one else can see them as I secretly enjoy this extra dimension, my jaw dropped in wonder.

* * *

My childhood friend and next-door neighbour, Danielle, comes to see me. We haven't seen each other for a couple of years, not since I left Manchester and moved to Bristol. She looks just the same with her mousy brown hair, pale blue eyes, and big smile. We used to go horse riding together when we were kids. Before we had horses of our own, we made reins out of belts that we attached to the handlebars of our bicycles and trotted around the village. I can't picture her fitting in with my media friends so I haven't invited her down to visit me. She doesn't drive on motorways, anyway. She rarely travels anywhere and has a simple life as a groom for a relatively rich woman who hunts.

It's good to see her. She's brought me a present, a colourful furry rooster. It's got flaps of red velvety fabric around its head and big chunky yellow legs that dangle off its plump body. I'm stunned because it's exactly the same soft toy I've just seen in the book that Kate sent me from Bristol. Kate, who also works at the Natural History Unit, the one who went out with Ella's boyfriend Jake for ten years. She sent me a Royal Photographic Society annual containing award-winning images from 1996. In one of the photos, there's a furry rooster sitting in a bird-cage with its legs dangling through the bars. It looks really sad. And here it is—the very same rooster—in the flesh! I'm pretty sure neither Kate nor Danielle is aware that my Chinese zodiac sign is rooster.

Apparently roosters are talkative, outspoken, frank, open, honest, and loyal individuals. We like to be the centre of attention and always appear attractive and beautiful. We are happiest when surrounded by others, whether at a party or just a social gathering, enjoying the spotlight.

Seeing these two identical roosters on the same day seems signifi-cant, though I don't exactly know why—maybe it has something to do with it waking everyone up in the morning. Some kind of wake-up call, perhaps. Like my psychosis is a wake-up call but *I'm* also a wake-up call to others—I'm here to wake people up.

Dinner arrives and I never know what the meal is going to be because I have to choose it so far in advance. Every day a form is given out with tomorrow's meal options. It's like a multiple-choice exam. I feel over-whelmed by the task of deciding what to eat so I usually let whoever's visiting me fill it in on my behalf. I hand Danielle the form giving her the responsibility. She's a bit nervous in case she chooses something I don't like.

'Don't worry, Danielle. It's all disgusting. Tick anything. It's just a game,' I reassure her.

Play the game. Take the meds. Be compliant. Act predictable. Look normal and get the hell out of here as soon as I can.

* * *

The consultants are finally here to see me. I go into their meeting room, the one the Mad Woman In The Attic was waiting outside. There are three of them with clipboards and pens. It feels intim-idating. They look buttoned up and stiff as boards. As far as I can remember, we've never met. I don't know who is who. They might all be consultants. Maybe two of them are students. They don't seem to think that my knowing is of any importance, because they don't introduce themselves.

'What's happened to me?' I ask, thinking they are the authority on me. One of them takes charge.

'As far as we can tell, you've had some kind of psychotic episode probably triggered by cannabis.' I blink at them blankly.

A psychotic episode? Triggered by cannabis? I'm in shock and can't fully take it in. They've never even asked me what I'm experiencing. Do they really think I'm psychotic? What about the angelic voice I heard? What about the auras? Aren't they going to ask me about those? This can't be right. I'm in deep denial.

'You'll need to be on anti-psychotic medication for at least six months.'

'Six months?' I'm incredulous. This is too much. The gap between their perception of who I am and who I feel myself to be is devastating. The emotion hits me like a train and I burst into tears, my in-breath desperately short, sharp, and trying to catch itself, like that of a six year old. No one offers me a tissue; there aren't even any in the room. Maybe nobody else cries in here. They're all too drugged up to feel anything. The consultants don't show any sign of emotion. They sit there waiting for me to finish. Then they ask me a question. They want to know, for their records, whether I heard any voices.

'Yes,' I reply, hoping they'll ask me more about it. But they don't. The woman just writes in her notes. They just wanted to confirm their diagnosis.

I'm a psycho.

* * *

I used to have romantic ideas about madness. It was always artists and poets who had a certain sensibility, their insanity portrayed as part of who they were. Nobody ever dwelled negatively on it because it's what gave them their genius. But I don't put myself in this category. My losing the plot feels like a shameful failure.

I don't question the diagnosis of the psychiatrists but deep down there's a niggling doubt about the cause. I think that whatever I've been through is probably the result of insomnia. Lack of sleep can make a person crazy, so I figure the psychosis was caused by me giving up cannabis and not by the drug itself. After all, I didn't start having strange apparitions until I had spent three nights without sleep. As soon as I recovered the lost sleep I was back to myself again.

I studied abnormal psychology as part of my degree and I was fascinated with the causes of schizophrenia, which is the label they give someone who is repeatedly psychotic. But the literature on the subject was conflicting. For the first two years we'd been learning about human development and how children affected by neglect, violence, sexual abuse, and other traumas often went on to suffer from mental health problems in later life. It seemed obvious to me why this would be. But in my final year we were given a very different picture during the Brain and Behaviour module. Suddenly everything was being explained from the perspective of neurological activity. It seemed that 'they' had discovered neurotransmitters that were the cause of schizophrenia: namely, dopamine. In a tutorial I expressed my confusion about the different theories. I couldn't understand why some people were saying that it was a social problem caused by childhood trauma but others claimed it was caused by chemical imbalances in the brain. I asked the tutor which one was correct. His response horrified me.

'I think the point is that we don't know.'

I felt ashamed at having asked the question and stupid for thinking he would have the answer. In fact, I was deeply troubled that he didn't. It meant I was studying a subject that we didn't really have a clue about. It was just different theories, and no certainty.

In 1996, only three years after studying abnormal psychology, and no closer to having any answers, I experienced a psychiatric system that operated as if it did know, and if you didn't agree with it you were seen as non-compliant, which only served as further evidence of your insanity.

CHAPTER FOUR

Discharge

D ad drives sedately through the urban sprawl of Greater Manchester. He's a much better driver since he semi-retired and stopped his stressful daily commute to the office. After my three weeks in hospital, he's pulled some strings, no doubt enjoying the challenge, to get me discharged. The red brick buildings are gloomy compared to the limestone around Bristol. The grey sky is oppressive as the moist air from the west coast hits the Pennines and rains often. But none of this matters to me because I'm free.

I lean my head against the car window watching the rhythm of the traffic flow in sync with the music on the stereo.

The Lighthouse Family serenades me and I am, as they say, lifted.

'Gifted, more like,' Dad jokes referring to all the get-well presents I've received. But I do feel lifted for a moment, lifted by the music, the perfect soundtrack to my journey back into the world.

* * *

I can't read because of the side effects of the medication. I can't concentrate on the words on the page. I can't type very well either because I don't have much muscle control of my fingers. I'm a bit stuck as to what to do. I'm bored. I got the sewing machine out today and made two skirts. Evenings bring relief that I've made it through another day.

Maybe a haircut will make me feel better, but I feel ashamed walking down to the village. The shuffling is embarrassing. At the hairdressers I don't like looking at myself in the mirror—my lips are really cracked and I'm skinny. The hairdresser tells me I look OK, but I know she's just being nice. I look like a shadow of my former self.

I have to visit the hospital every week. I complain about the medication and its side effects. Apparently I'm very sensitive to it. They suggest changing it to Sulpiride but that turns out to be even worse than Haloperidol. Both my legs freeze up from shaking so fast. Dad massages them as I lie on the sofa but it's unbearable. I can't do this for six months.

'Why don't you stop taking it?' Dad suggests.

'Stop taking the medication?' I'm surprised he's going against the advice of the psychiatric profession. 'What do you think, Mum?' Mum agrees. I feel relieved and it gives me permission and the confidence to go against the advice of the medical profession. The doctor says if I stop taking it then next time it will take longer to get better and the tablets won't work as well.

What kind of medication is that? And next time? There's not going to be a next time. His fear tactics fail to manipulate me.

* * *

I'm standing at the doorway to the reunion with my soul. A stranger approaches and I tell him I want to have faith again.

'If you want to have faith again,' he says, 'you have to put these underpants on your head and breathe deeply.' He's holding up a pair of old stained Y-fronts. 'You might die. But then you will be reunited with your soul. On the other hand you might live and then you'll have faith again.' I put the smelly-looking pants over my head, feeling silly and a little apprehensive. I bravely take a deep breath in through my nose. The odour is neutral and not unpleasant at all. It was just a ruse to see how far I would go.

I haven't realised I've not been dreaming until I wake up feeling exhilarated from this powerful one this morning. For the first time in ages I feel glad to be alive, clearer and cleaner somehow. The clamps have come off my brain. My vision is no longer cloudy and my muscles are my own again. I know for a fact it's from stopping taking the antipsychotics.

* * *

A small parcel arrives from Solomon, a demo tape of his latest album I asked him to send. I see the word 'fear' written on the sleeve. I blink and look again. My mind is playing tricks on me. It says 'Feet', the name of his band. There's a letter with it, which is hard to read because of the messy handwriting.

Sol
Bristol
Monday
Late
Dear M,

Cool ... I'm glad you rang ... as I said I wasn't too sure with regard to the ol' phonage.
Twas all a bit of a shock to hear about you ... but you were wiped out when you came into M.A.S.H. and 'bit' is an understatement!
I hope you manage to kick all this shit into check ... as I'm sure you will ...
Is your work seeing you right, and how about the flat? ...
I tried to claim invalidity benefit and the DHSS said I was a slack git cuz I ain't paid nuff N.I. Still the tax man can take a flyer as I've come clean and am about to wedge him up.
On the tape tip ... The album as it stands is on one side and a little jammy bit on the 'B' ... but the rest of the stuff is old stuff I found on record that we'd put together earlier ... à la Blue Peter circa 92 ...
I'll send you some new stuff that we're workin on now. Odd jazz beats not for the faint hearted.

He's drawn a heart, which he's shaded in on one side so it looks lit from the other. Beneath it he's written the word 'Boomerang' with a question mark.
    'What are your current feelings about Bristol? Do you think you've had it?' the letter continues. Does he mean Bristol or him? I'm always reading between the lines and over-analysing. Why the heart doodle?

Is the word boomerang next to the heart asking me if I'm coming back to him?

I put his album on and listen for clues there, any mention of me. The trip hop Bristol beats sound eerie and disturbing and set my heart racing.

Was that 'Emma's eyes' I just heard him sing?

Oooooh oooh I can see through you.

You're invisible, not visible.

Does he mean me? He can see through me?

I'm all jittery. My belly is quivering and I feel quite wobbly. I switch it off and throw the cassette into the bedside table. I can't listen; it's doing my head in. I think I have to let this one go. I need to be with someone who can communicate properly.

* * *

Mum puts a cup of tea for me on the kitchen table and sits down opposite. She's stroking her mug awkwardly like she has something difficult to say.

'Do you remember what you said in the hospital about being sexually abused?' Mum's probably rehearsed this sentence in her head. It's one of those awkward mother and daughter conversations we don't find easy. Like when she asked me how much I knew about sex or whether the relationship with my first proper boyfriend had become 'physical'. I do remember something vaguely about thinking I had been sexually abused.

'Yes,' I reply monosyllabically, not making it any easier for her.

'Is it true?' Mum asks.

'No. I don't know why I said it,' I tell her. She looks relieved but still awkward.

'Well. Er. I spoke to Sally about it. To see if she knew anything. I asked your sister if she had any idea why you might have mentioned it.'

'And?' I ask. Mum composes herself before speaking.

'She said that the *gardien* in Abidjan sexually abused her. She's never told anyone about it. Do you know anything about this? Do you remember anything?'

'The *gardien*? The man that was supposed to guard the house? That's ironic. No. I didn't know anything.'

I remember a man, who I thought was the gardener for some reason, playing with us outside on the patio. We played what I've always called the bean game but that's probably not its real name.

The counters were made of massive, shiny, grey beans, the kind you probably only get in Africa. The board was wooden and hand carved, hollowed out to make eight holes on each player's side. The game started with the beans being placed in sets of four in each compartment. The idea was to win as many beans as possible by choosing which pile to start from. A turn consisted of selecting a pile, dropping a bean consecutively into each hollowed out bowl until you only had one left. If that landed in an empty hole your turn was over but if it landed in a hollow with other beans then you got to pick those up and continue around. When it landed with three other beans then you made a four, which you kept. The person with the most beans at the end was the winner. The skill was in counting back from a pile of three to see if you could find one that would make you land there thus making it a four. My sister and I used to play it for hours. But we got a different pleasure from it. We felt the most glee landing on the biggest pile of beans that had built up during the course of the game. Our small five- and six-year-old hands couldn't hold so many at once so we actually had to use two hands. When that happened, the look on the other's face was priceless: envy to the max. That was the real winning!

So the man we played that game with was sexually abusing her? I wonder why she never told anyone before.

I take a sip of tea and sense the conversation is over.

* * *

I'm finally back in Bristol to see if I can sneak back into my old life. Minus the drugs. I've been moaning about the boredom of being at my parents' house but down here, with everyone busy working, I feel redundant. I'm on my own in the flat all day with nothing to do. Without work, I'm at a loose end. Ella spends most of her free time with Jake now, so I hardly hang out with her. Sol and Zanna are now officially an item so I avoid that whole crowd too. Without the drugs, it's no fun hanging out with them anyway. I need to find some new friends.

Claire and Chris, who rescued me, have been in touch. They've asked me to do some mystery shopping for them. They run a customer services business that Claire's dad started. He used to run a pub, which is how Claire and Chris met. They both worked there when they were eighteen. Her dad used all his pub contacts to start a new enterprise. Claire and Chris have expanded it to include retail outlets and apparently they're doing really well. I've been a mystery shopper for them before, when we were students, which was basically just going to the pub for free. It's not much money but I appreciate their thinking of me. I think they're just trying to help, plus it will give me something to do.

People are being very sweet to me. I'm not used to all the concern and it's a bit embarrassing. A friend at work, Paul, has asked me to help out on a shoot for a programme he's working on. It's just a few days as a runner. It ruffled my feathers a bit taking running work after being a researcher but I didn't want to seem ungrateful. I like Paul. He's friendly and sensitive and has been having a hard time with a break-up so I won't have to put on any kind of happy front.

It feels strange going back there after what's happened. I don't know who knows what. I know Mum told my boss I had a breakdown, but people might have heard about my diagnosis through Ella. No one mentions it but the *how are yous?* are loaded with awkwardness and sympathetic concern. I don't want them to know, and I don't want to be labelled psychotic.

The word 'psychotic' has got to be one of the most shocking in the English language. When I use it to let people know what I've been through, it often leads to a strange reaction. People don't know what to say because it's more than they are able to deal with. The word gets a little stuck in my throat but I overcompensate and use it more widely than I'm comfortable with. I think it might be a fucked-up form of protest.

I'm introduced to Ovid Star, Paul's director, and I'm nervous. He launches straight into having been through his own dark night of the soul and I don't know what to say. I feel all shades of awkward, but he seems like a nice guy. He sounds American and has greasy, black, curly hair. He looks like he's lived an interesting life and I've no idea where he's suddenly appeared from. People come and go like that in TV, chasing a contract anywhere they can get it. It's not a very stable life and attracts wild and flamboyant, artistic types.

The studio is in a big industrial space in Easton and I'm on call to run errands. In the dressing room my friend Paul, who's the researcher, is having his body painted gold. He's meant to be a Greek god and is doing a pretty good impression of one. He's so good-looking they don't have to hire a model, and he's got one of those dimples in his chin that makes him look like Timothy Dalton.

I'm told to head off in the van to get some supplies. I'm a bit flustered driving a strange vehicle in a part of town I don't really know. It's a big van and I don't even have a car so I'm out of practice. I can't see shit out of the back and as soon as I reverse I hear the unmistakable sound of metal crunching and feel the bumper squishing like butter. My face flushes and I get out to inspect the damage. It's not so bad, but I don't like having to tell Ovid; I don't want him to think I'm a liability. He's actually fine about it when I break the news. It's only a hire car, and that's what insurance is for.

I think it's going to take me a while to get back into this whole TV thing. I've lost all my confidence.

* * *

I make my way to Temple Meads and get the next train to Cardiff. Today I'm a mystery shopper. The hi-fi store is easy to find and I walk in feeling unsure of myself. I don't really know how I'm supposed to act but I can't exactly be honest because that would give the game away. The deceit feels awkward. I'm not interested in buying a new stereo and have no idea what to look for. I've been told to buy something 'bottom of the range'. I want to look like a genuine customer, but I just can't be bothered to get into the finer details of stereo technology. Eventually an assistant comes to my rescue.

'Can I help at all?'

'I'm looking for a stereo. Not too expensive.' He leads the way and points at a shelf.

'These are all reasonably priced.'

'I don't really know about stereos.' I look confused by the rows of identical, black, rectangular shaped stacks.

'This one is good for the price,' the assistant encourages.

'Great, I'll take it.' No one buys anything that quickly—I should have asked more questions. They'll know I'm not a genuine customer.

I pay by card and leave with a big box under my arm. On the train home I fill in the form asking questions about points of my encounter that I didn't really take any notice of, or have an opinion about. I should have looked at the form before I went in, but I just decide to be nice, and give them a glowing report.

Walking back to my flat, I feel like something's missing. I steer my mind towards thinking about where I've just been, and what I was doing there—and realise I'm supposed to be carrying a box. Damn! I've left the stereo on the train. *What an idiot! I've fucked up again.* How am I going to explain this to Claire and Chris?

I get back to my flat and immediately call the local police station.

'I'd like to report a robbery,' I lie. The police officer takes my details: name, address, and telephone number.

'So, tell me what happened,' he says.

'I was walking down Blackboy Hill about half an hour ago when a shortish guy with a shaved head walked past me and snatched the box from under my arm and ran away.' I'm imagining it happening outside Sol's flat, and I describe Solomon without giving too many precise details. I don't want him to be falsely accused but I do need to give a description, and he's all I can think of.

'This is quite a serious matter. Would you be able to come in to the station to make a statement?' I wasn't expecting that. I've presumed that there is so much crime, they won't actually have time to investigate most of it. They never do anything about my £500 bike that gets stolen at least once a year, so I'm surprised a cheap stereo has caused such alarm.

'Er. Yeah. OK.' We make an appointment for me to come into the station. I've dug myself into quite a hole, so I call Claire and tell her what's happened.

'It's all right, Emma. It's probably still on the train. Where was the train going?' Claire takes charge of the situation.

'Taunton, I think.'

'If you call Taunton station they'll be able to check it. Hopefully it'll be exactly where you left it and they'll put it on the next train back to Bristol.' Why didn't I think of that?

The stereo is still on the train when it pulls into the station and it's escorted back to Bristol just as Claire said. Now I just have the embarrassing task of explaining to the police.

* * *

I've been officially discharged from the hospital's system up north and a letter arrives inviting me to register with the psychiatric department down here. I have to wait ages in the waiting room for the appointment, which I think is a complete waste of time. There's nothing wrong with me now so why do I have to go through all this?

A woman in a white lab style coat comes for me and leads me into a small office. It's bare and not very personal so probably belongs to no one in particular. We sit opposite each other at a desk and she takes a clipboard out of the drawer. She reads the questions without looking at me and writes on it as I answer. She asks me about my life, my childhood, and my education.

'Were you sexually abused as a child?' I wasn't expecting that question. It's like she's trying to build up a profile of me to satisfy the diagnosis.

'No,' I tell her. I'm not one of those cases. She'll have to find another explanation for my psychosis. Then she asks me about drug taking. I see no reason to hide anything. I tell her I don't use drugs any more but have taken the occasional class A, recreationally: ecstasy, speed, LSD, cocaine but never heroin or crack. I tell her I smoked cannabis every day for about seven years. That seems to satisfy her curiosity.

I'm an open-and-shut case of cannabis psychosis.

* * *

Making my way to the police station, I'm going through in my head what I'm going to say. My appointment is at Southmead; I don't know why. It's not my local area nor anywhere near where I claim the robbery took place. But apparently robbery is a serious police matter and much worse than normal theft.

It's a quiet place with very little going on. I've an appointment with the detective inspector. I think he knows I made up the story, and that's probably why he's called me in: to call my bluff. There's probably something glaringly obvious about it that gives me away. I really wasn't expecting all this fuss; it's only a stereo, and a cheap one at that.

I open the door leading to his office and take the seat that's offered. The detective inspector is not in uniform, which makes me feel a little less nervous, but my hands are still clammy and I'm finding it hard to speak. He clicks his pen on and off a few times while he looks at a form on his desk in front of him. It's a large desk and it looks antique, solid compared to the rest of the décor, the institutionalised linoleum floor and tatty, old, off-white walls. He looks up at me and begins:

'Thanks for coming into the station. I'd like to find out more about the robbery that took place on Blackboy Hill on—'

'I've got a confession to make,' I blurt out, interrupting. 'There wasn't a robbery.'

'There wasn't a robbery?'

'No. I made it up. I'm really sorry.'

'You made it up?'

'I left the stereo on the train. I forgot all about it because it wasn't really mine. I only bought it because I was a mystery shopper for my friend's company, and I totally forgot about it when I got off the train. I didn't want to tell my friend because I thought she would think I didn't really care. I thought if I got a police report then she would be able to account for it and never need know. But I didn't realise robbery was such a serious matter. I'm really sorry for wasting police time.'

'Right,' he says looking serious. 'My colleague is just preparing the gallows for you out the back.' For a split second, his humour doesn't register. He's a policeman after all. Then my anxiety gives way to relief.

* * *

So I've succeeded in giving up cannabis, having followed through with my determination to do so, even though it led to a psychiatric hospitalisation. To support myself to remain drug-free, I change my circle of friends and try to put the whole episode behind me. I don't look too deeply into the causes because I think it won't happen again. Now the dope is out of my system I can get to sleep no problem so there's no reason to think I'll have another episode. But one of the nurses in the hospital told my Mum that the psychosis would either disappear as quickly as it arrived, or it would return again and again. Six years later, in February 2003, it does exactly that.

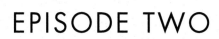

EPISODE TWO

CHAPTER FIVE

New Zealand

A lot has changed. My home, my job, and my friends. First, I move into a shared house with three other girls who also work in telly. Jess knows everyone because she's really friendly. Pippa's into similar outdoor sports as me and Jane is just all-round lovely, soft and caring. They don't do drugs but they still know how to have fun. It's like an episode of *Sex and the City*. Loads of people came to my thirtieth birthday celebration thanks to Jess's connections and the house's reputation as a media party house.

It's a Victorian terrace with huge bay windows in Clifton Wood, perched on a hill near two elaborate Georgian crescents. I cycle through Clifton Village every morning to the independent production company where I work—thanks to a presenter I met at the BBC.

We both worked on the same series a while ago and he managed to get his own show on Channel 5. The company has never done any wildlife documentaries before so they asked him if he knew of any good researchers. For some reason he mentioned me. He probably doesn't know about my mental health history. I think he just fancies me.

This job has taken me on some amazing trips around the world: filming leatherback turtles laying eggs on a beach in Costa Rica; diving in a cage with great white sharks in South Africa; tracking unhabituated gorillas in Uganda. We also filmed vampire bats in Costa Rica. We were halfway down a kilometre-long, disused railway tunnel when we heard a noise. It sounded like the Severn Bore coming around the corner. Then I remembered that the Severn Bore, which I'd gone to see for my thirtieth birthday, had itself sounded like a train coming. *Shit, there's a train!* In a split second I had to make a decision about whether to run, with a very heavy battery over my shoulder, or dive into the alcove where the vampire bats were roosting. The rest of the crew ran, so I followed them. I was pretty sure I was dead. I kept turning around to shine the light behind me so the driver would see us and slow down. Ten metres or so from the entrance, there was a huge puddle. My wellies filled up with water and felt like lead boots, and the energy drained from me. I called out for help and our driver and guide rushed in, and carried me the last few feet. When the train passed by, it was going at a snail's pace. Two men stuck their toothless, grinning heads out of the window, laughing like cartoon villains. We drank ourselves silly that night, replaying the events over to each other, to get over the trauma.

After researching that series, they asked me to direct. I couldn't believe it. *I'm a director!* How did that happen? I did some directing at the BBC, but only the odd short piece for a magazine show. I directed Chris Packham at the red kite feeding centre in Wales. It was a straightforward enough story: in presenter-led wildlife shoots, it's all about the two-shot. You have to get the celebrity and the animal in the same shot, to prove they were really there. With wild animals it's tricky, because they invariably scarper when there's any humans about. Luckily, at a feeding centre, it was easy. They see humans all the time, in the hides, putting out meat for them. It all went well until I got back to the office where I got a tongue-lashing for not having put any make-up on Chris. Apparently he had a spot on his upper lip, which I hadn't thought necessary to hide. It's not something I care about; I don't wear make-up! But the series producer was annoyed that I didn't cover it up—he said I should have put make-up over it.

I've also got myself a boyfriend. On my way up the hill one morning, a guy I vaguely recognise is walking down. He works as a researcher with my housemate Jane and he gets a lift with her to the office. He has striking, tightly curled brown hair and clear, pale blue eyes. As we pass, I get this odd sensation of already knowing him, though I don't think we've ever spoken.

'Hello,' I say.

'Hello,' he says back, and then goes on his way. I rack my brains for the memory of an earlier meeting but can't find one.

At the next party, fancy dress with a Bond theme, I put on a pair of tight shorts and my rock climbing harness, ready to abseil down a sky-scraper, cut a hole through the window, dodge the criss-crossing alarm sensors and break into a safe.

I see him again across the other side of the room. He's looking right at me, and an impulse takes me. I strut across the dance floor in my long, lace-up, brown leather boots and we don't take our eyes off each other the whole way. He takes my hand and leads me outside into an alley where he kisses me like a teenager. He's only twenty-three, seven years younger than me, but the age gap feels irrelevant. His name is Oscar.

I also get £5,000 in compensation for being knocked off my bike when a car door opens across the cycle lane, breaking the scaphoid bone in my hand. Enough for a deposit on a house. So I move again, into my own home this time, a pink cottage in Bishopston, just off the Gloucester Road, which is a thriving high street with lots of independent shops and cafés. I'm the first of my friends to buy, but they're all following suit now—Jane and Jess and others—getting on the property ladder.

It's terrifying at first, the idea of having a mortgage. I get a lodger, to take the pressure off, and he's now going to rent the whole place out with his girlfriend whilst I go off to New Zealand. I always planned on visiting the country again after our family had a holiday there, touring around in a motorhome. You can get a work visa for a year up until the age of thirty so I got one just before I reached the cut-off point. Oscar looked hurt when I first mentioned it, but there's nothing stopping him from joining me.

I don't have a master plan for my travels. I just need to get away. I feel restless and a little dissatisfied with working in television. I'm chuffed to be a director so early on in my career but I don't particularly care for the programmes I make. Many wildlife shows focus on hunt-ing, killing, and violent attacks and it's only the big sexy animals that get a look in. It's not just the emphasis on violence that bothers me. It's the avoidance of more important issues that I believe we should be showing the world. Television has the power to affect change and I think we should be broadcasting films about the state of the planet due to man's influence: climate change, species extinctions, and habitats dis-appearing. But these subjects are apparently 'doom and gloom' and not what the viewers want. Films about sharks and Nazis are no-brainers, guaranteed to attract audiences.

Quite a few of my media friends are also feeling the same. A couple of them have even branched out into holistic therapy—Bristol is quite an 'alternative' city. They've been doing shiatsu courses and regularly use me as a body to practise on. Now I want to have a proper, full length, professional treatment so I book myself in for a session with a therapist who comes highly recommended by my friends.

The shiatsu practitioner is petite, dressed in crisp, white, loose clothes and hair in a tight ballet dancer's bun.

'Have you had shiatsu before?'

'I've had a ten minute taster and some treatments from friends who were training, but that's it.'

'And why are you here?'

'I just want to see what it's like.' She doesn't try to force me to say any more than that. I'm glad because I'm not really sure why I'm there. Since that first taster session I've been curious about shiatsu.

Shiatsu means 'finger pressure' in Japanese. It is based on the same principles as acupuncture but without the needles. Energy, or chi, flows through all things and when it gets blocked, through injury, repeated tension, or repressing emotions, the body gets sick. Symptoms are seen as a warning light that something is wrong. Shiatsu uses touch, pressure, and manipulative techniques to rebalance the flow of chi so that the body heals itself and then the symptom disappears. This is completely at odds with the Western view of symptoms as being things to get rid of. If you have a headache, for example, you take a painkiller but it doesn't actually address the underlying cause.

I lie on the futon mattress on the floor and the practitioner quietly and swiftly makes her way around me. It's not like the vigorous pummelling of the taster session. She's gentle and often stays in one place for a while before moving on. Her touch is delicate and loving.

She rests her fingers tenderly on my chest. My face flushes and I feel uncomfortable. Emotions I don't recognise are creeping up to the surface. My mind starts racing. She's really close to my breasts. This feels too intimate. Oh God, what if she thinks I'm a lesbian? This is the most vulnerable I've ever felt and I don't like it. It's totally unfamiliar.

At the end of the session she takes a small hand towel and rolls it up. She wedges it under my spine, the weight of my body pushing open my torso at the front. She doesn't explain why it needs opening, but I trust her when she tells me to do it at home on a regular basis.

I make my way back to my place, on foot, past the busy rush hour traffic. The wide pavements are crammed with people. I think about what I'll have for dinner and whether I need to buy anything. I don't feel like shopping right now, so I decide to make do with whatever's in the fridge.

A ripple of something rises up through my chest and my eyes fill with tears. I keep walking, hoping it will subside but the damn bursts. I'm properly crying in broad daylight, my face screwed up with muffled sobs, which are actually fully audible. I hold my head upright, composed, trying not to draw any attention to myself, and nobody seems to notice. There's no doubt in my mind the shiatsu has unleashed all this and there's little I can do to stop it, so I just let the tears flow.

* * *

It's a two-day bus ride from Auckland to Wanaka. I'm tired from rushing around jet-lagged, sending off CVs to all the TV production companies in the city. I've got myself a New Zealand mobile but I'm not expecting any calls for work soon and I can't get out of the rat race fast enough. I'm heading to the mountains of the South Island for the rest of the ski season, to do some snowboarding. It's good to finally stop and let the world pass by through the coach window rather than having to go out and get it.

Headphones on, I'm tuned into a local radio station. Apart from the accent, there's little to differentiate it from any commercial stations back in the UK. Most of the songs are the same with similar over-the-top adverts. It's the soundtrack to my journey and I'm enjoying it, even though it's mostly cheesy pop.

I watch the landscape change from an urban sprawl of tropical, palm tree-lined avenues to lush, green hills and volcanic peaks.

Ronan Keating's na na nas catch me off guard with a jingly boyband beat, making my bus ride feel like a music video. Cut to a close-up in my head of the bus wheel spinning. Then an image of Oscar walking down a big, open highway, arms wide apart singing to camera like Ronan.

The lyrics tug at my heart. I've come halfway around the world to hear the UK's No.1 tell me that I've found love. My throat tightens up.

I wipe away the tears from my now wet cheeks and reach for the photo of Oscar in my purse. I miss him already.

* * *

Once the winter season is over, I head to Dunedin to stay with an old school friend, Dave, who used to sit next to me in GCSE history in Hong Kong. I did get offered some TV work in Auckland. My mobile rang whilst I was on a ski lift. The series was a reality show where contestants were given NZ$500 to invest. I couldn't face working on something that was all about making money so I turned it down with the excuse that I'd just spent two days on a bus and didn't feel like going all the way back to Auckland so soon.

Dave got in touch with me a while ago though Friends Reunited and very kindly said I could stay with him as long as I liked. He lives in a detached Victorian house up on the hill above Dunedin. The air is crisp and clean and I could like it if I wasn't so homesick.

I get a job at a café on the Octagon, the main square in town. They make me maître d' after my first shift and I enjoy the buzz. I'm good at waiting tables. I smile a lot, I'm friendly and attentive to the customers. I keep an eye on the orders and what stage they're at. *Do their plates need clearing? Do they need the bill?* I'm conscientious and don't hang around chatting like the others. I'm always on the go, and if there's nothing to do, I stand at the counter rolling the clean cutlery into paper napkins. The staff is pretty much my only social life, apart from Dave. Dave always cracked me up at school. We had a lot of fun in class, but his carefree attitude seems to have been squeezed out of him in his pursuit of work. He works for Mercedes and though he's not quite in the twenty-first century with email and computers, he has got slightly lost in the everyday stresses of life. He doesn't seem to have any hobbies except pootling around in a mint-condition classic car—a Mercedes, of course. He looks after his garden at the weekends and drinks a lot of beer. His kitchen is the least lived-in room in the house, in contrast to his front lounge with its leather chairs and expensive sound system, where he sits for hours listening to The Beatles.

Every day, when I'm not on a shift, I make a point of spending time lying on a rolled up tea towel, like the shiatsu practitioner showed me. It really does open my chest and it makes me cry. I miss Oscar but I think these tears are older than that. Tears I buried a long time ago.

I explore the coastline of the Otago Peninsular, which juts out from Dunedin. The hills are remnants of an extinct volcano. I make my way up to the top of a lookout point and perch precariously on a rocky outcrop. The water below is crystal clear and in the distance, where it gets deeper, it reflects the turquoise sky. A seal is swimming only a few metres away from the edge. I've got a bird's eye view as it bends and swirls gracefully. It's mesmerising.

I'm a water baby and practically grew up in the sea. When we lived in the Ivory Coast we went to the beach on Sundays and spent all day in the waves, which seemed huge, relative to my little four-year-old body. They lifted my feet off the ground, spun me around like a washing machine. My bikini bottoms used to fill up with sand until I dropped them in the next wave to clear them out. At the end of the day we had to pick off the thick, black, oil that had got stuck to the bottom of our feet. Ignorant of the oil fields out at sea, I thought this was entirely normal, just how beaches were.

The seal moves around in circles and figures of eight. This mammal is perfectly adapted for hunting underwater, in sharp contrast to the way it lollops about on land. Its dark, curved shape twists and turns, agile and free. Oblivious to my human eyes, it touches something deep in my soul and speaks to the hidden, feminine force inside me, as yet dormant but waiting to be unleashed.

* * *

The best thing about New Zealand is the tramping. There are loads of four-day hikes that provide huts equipped with bunk beds so you don't have to carry a tent. You can also refill your water bottles, keeping your pack weight right down. I've done lots of them. Sometimes on my own, sometimes with visiting family or friends. Oscar did his back in so hasn't managed to make it here, but we're still in touch. Probably just as well—he hates walking anyway, and never once joined me on hikes in England.

I'm stomping along at a pace that doesn't allow time to take in any of the idyllic, wild mountainous surroundings of Mount Aspiring National Park. I've got one focus and one focus only: to get to the hut before nightfall. I couldn't find the start of this tramp; faffed about for ages trying to wade across the wrong part of the Makarora River. It turned out there were two places with the same name right next to each other so it was an easy mistake to make. I've now got five hours of daylight to walk a seven-hour route. I'm on the right track at least and the path is wide and obvious.

The sun sets early behind the mountains and the wooded trail shades what little light there is. I have a torch, but I don't know how long the battery will last or how far I still have to go so I'm not sure about using it. As the last of the light dims, my heart quickens and panic sets in. The forest is dense and I can't see the path in front of me. My breathing is shallow and my head feels bent with fear. There's no point hurrying now so I stop to calm myself down with a talking-to.

I'm in New Zealand. There are no dangerous beasts here, not like in Australia. It's just dark. The trail is wide and safe; I must stay on it at all costs. The only danger is straying off the path. I have a torch and I must use it and risk running out of battery. If that happens I can sleep on the footpath. I have a sleeping bag and it's not that cold. But losing the trail in this wilderness could mean death. *So stop panicking and switch the torch on!*

The beam lights up small reflectors I hadn't seen before that have been nailed onto the trees to mark the way. I flash ahead of me briefly then switch the torch off to save power. Then I walk a short distance before flicking it on again to get my next bearing. I feel calmed, grateful for these night-time waymarkers.

The path opens to a river, which lets in a little moonlight. I walk along its true left bank, upstream and uphill until I come to a crossing. This time there's a wooden bridge, small but sturdy. On the other side there's a T-junction in the trail. Turning right is the most logical thing to do, to continue walking upstream rather than left and back on myself. But I get a weird feeling and without thinking, my feet take me left, like an invisible sign is pointing that way. Downstream the woods open out to a small clearing and there ahead of me is the hut. I made it!

I spend the night on one of the top bunks, the only person there. In the morning I track back to the bridge, taking the path to the right, which I luckily didn't take yesterday. It leads to a high pass, cold and exposed. If I'd taken this last night, I would have overshot my overnight stay and perished in the cold. The thought stirs something inside me I don't understand and I'm afraid it might rearrange my whole world view. I have a feeling it was my grandmother telling me which way to go. I don't believe in life after death and wonder how I'm going to explain this to Oscar when we see each other again. He doesn't believe in that kind of spiritual crap either.

My parents didn't bring me up into any religion. Dad believed in us being allowed to make our own choices and Mum thought that religion was the cause of many of the world's problems. I wasn't one of those children who saw dead people or fairies either. I loved the magic of Walt Disney's fairytales but that was that. They weren't real and I could tell the difference. I took great pleasure in finding out that Father Christmas was just Mum hiding toys in a secret cupboard. I had zero interest in spirituality and didn't have the time or inclination to contemplate the meaning of life because my head was stuffed full of the school syllabus.

After my A Levels, when I was taking a year off from the education system, I finally had time to read whatever I felt liked. I found myself devouring books about spiritual subjects: *Life After Life* by Raymond Moody; *Afterlife* by Colin Wilson; books about psychics and mediums like Edgar Cayce and Shirley MacLaine's memoirs *Going Within* and *It's All in the Playing*. I was fascinated by the supernatural encounters Shirley described having at Machu Pichu in Peru.

All these books pointed to us having a consciousness that continued after death. They also talked about how we can receive help from those not currently in physical form because there is actually no death: it's just a shedding of the body. I also explored Buddhism, and the idea of enlightenment as being achievable in this lifetime appealed. It was all very heady and I didn't put any of it into practice, but I did feel a longing to experience something magical.

When my Mum said she thought Shirley MacLaine's latest book *Out on a Limb* was contrived, I felt myself close down, shrinking back to the narrow confines of my mortal body. My ego climbed back into the spiritual closet and shut the door.

Then, at university, I got the impression the academic world thought there was nothing beyond the material and scientifically measurable. Spiritual beliefs were for people who needed a crutch. Uni taught me to be critical and I adopted a cynicism to go with it, like driving around in a tank. I was highly educated, therefore I was an atheist and I hid my spiritual interests so well that I eventually forgot about them.

This experience in New Zealand was a very quiet, intuitive feeling that woke up these old questions and stirred the spiritual passion I had buried. If it *was* my grandmother guiding me then it meant a part of us *did* survive beyond death. If that was true then there was a lot more to this world than I'd allowed myself to believe.

* * *

The tenants in my house in Bristol hand in their notice, giving me an excuse to go back to the UK. I'm tired of missing Oscar and am happy to be leaving two months earlier than planned. On my return, I soon broach the subject of spirituality with him.

'What would you do if I started believing in God?' I ask, opting for the worst-case scenario of my recent spiritual questioning. His face explodes like an animation, his eyes popping out as he coughs and splutters.

'God?' He spits the word out. It's too incredible for him to get his head around. Emma, the cynical, sceptical, level-headed mocker of superstitious nonsense? Emma, the scientist-respecting, evolutionary psychologist who reads books like *The Rise and Fall of the Third Chimpanzee*? I know how he perceives the idea of God because I've seen it that way too. I don't believe in God either but I no longer have an aversion to the concept. I've become an agnostic, not an atheist. I want the freedom to explore, stay open to the possibility, in a safe and tolerant environment. I don't want to close down again because of other people's attitudes. But Oscar's reaction is the beginning of the end of our relationship.

CHAPTER SIX

Union

I probably stand out like a country bumpkin in London. I tell myself no one is looking at me. They're all too busy in their own heads but I'm worried I'm not wearing the right clothes. I'm shivering with the February cold and interview nerves. Work has been harder to find since I came back from New Zealand. I don't like this freelancing lifestyle, living from one short contract to the next. I'm having to explore my plan B—getting a job in London.

The offices are spacious with high ceilings and minimalist white-washed walls. I'm greeted politely by an assistant and led to a small meeting room where a man and a woman are waiting for me. They sit next to each other on one side of a table and usher me towards the chair on the opposite side. After some small talk about my journey there, the interview begins in earnest.

They take it in turns to tell me about the new series I would be working on and how the company loves to do things differently. It's a travel show but they want to shoot it in a whole new stylised way. They're looking for cutting-edge directors with original ideas.

'We'd like to film the presenter in really creative ways,' the man explains. 'If you were directing a piece to camera about sailing for example, how would you do it differently?' My brain freezes. I hate being asked for ideas on the spot. I can never think of any under pressure but I have to answer the question so I just give him an obvious one.

'I'd probably shoot them on a jetty with yachts in the background.'

'That's not very creative,' he snaps irritated. I feel stupid and I want to get out. I don't want to work with this guy.

'I really loved the way you filmed the tree bark piece in your showreel,' the woman rescues me, playing good cop to his bad. 'It was quirky and stylish. Why don't you think more along those lines.' Her encouragement gives me the confidence I need. Suddenly I see an image of water droplets on a sheet of glass, then pulling focus to reveal the presenter, the now-blurred drops of water making beautiful prism shapes in the foreground.

I can't tell if they like it or not as they're both poker-faced. Without any feedback I feel vulnerable. Maybe they think I'm crazy.

When the interview is over I head back on the train to Bristol. I don't really want to move to London but I've been doing a lot of temping work in-between contracts and sometimes it's six months before another TV job comes along. I hate being freelance: the insecurity, always having to be on the lookout for the next opportunity.

Back home my lodger is watching TV so I plonk myself down in the armchair and join him. I don't normally watch *Who Wants to Be a Millionaire?*—I'm not into game shows, but I want the lodger to feel like it's his home too, so the living room is now a place of compromise. If he's there first, then I watch what he's watching.

The camera pans across the contestants who are sitting in a long row, waiting for the opportunity to compete for a place in the chair.

'Put these kings into the order in which they were on the throne,' Chris Tarrant barks. The editor cuts from one face to another. Music creates obvious tension for the audience and lights flash, letting us know when someone's completed the task.

'Who's next in the hot seat?' Chris teases.

'It's him,' I say to my lodger Nigel, pointing as the shot pans past Andrew Fairfax from Norwich. Maybe he looks the fastest or the most determined. I don't know *how* I know. I just know. It *feels* like it's going to be him.

'Andrew Fairfax from Norwich!' Chris declares.

'Wow. How weird is that? I *knew* it was going to be him!'

'Just a lucky guess,' says Nigel, not in the least bit impressed by my sudden precognitive abilities. I can't be bothered to argue with him. He's a film studies lecturer with a PhD in cynicism.

A few days later I've got another interview. It's much more laid-back, at a company I've already worked for in Bristol, but it's still nerve-wracking. I pretend to sound interested in the series but the truth is I'm not. It's another violent portrayal of dangerous wildlife in an attempt to get high viewing figures and the idea of actually working on it makes me lose the will to live. All I can think of to say is 'sharks' and 'Nazis' so I mostly keep quiet.

When the interview is over, I cycle home to relax in my little pink house, a sanctuary within the city. With two interviews in one week, I feel quite stressed out. My nerves are jangly and all my actions are speedy, like a wind-up toy.

I lie on my bed and rest my hands on my belly, feeling the gentle rising and falling of my breath. The interviews play back in my mind. Neither of them went that well, as I didn't take the initiative to sell myself. I let out a sigh, yawning slightly. My palms are quite hot. Not sweaty on the outside but a lovely warmth coming from inside them and into my body like the vapour from Aladdin's lamp. Something is pouring out of my hands and winding its way through me. My body is responding; my right hip loosening; my left buttock dropping. I keep my hands in the same place until it feels done and then move them to a different position. I don't really know what I'm doing but it's smoothing out the cracks.

I've no idea how long I've been doing this for. It's getting dark so it must be about five o'clock, which means I've been here for several hours. I break contact and sit up. An empty picture frame I've not yet found a photo for, that's leaning against the wall, catches my attention. Looking into the centre of it, the dark rectangle where a colourful image should be, I'm pulled in. I stare into the blackness.

Nothingness.

The void.

From nothingness and nowhere comes a thought.

Oh my God, I'm going to die!

My breath freezes as my diaphragm jams up. I turn round to face the bed, then jolt backwards.

I don't want to die in my bed.

Then I remember six years ago talking about death to Claire on the phone and somehow I make the connection. It's happening again.

I don't want to be alone, so I call my now ex-boyfriend, Oscar. He laughs at the idea that I'm going to die but comes over immediately.

'Will you stay the night just to keep an eye on me?'

'OK. If you want me to, but you're not going to die.'

'What if I die in the night? They might think you're responsible.'

'Who's *they*?' he asks.

'The police.'

'The police?' Oscar thinks for a second. 'Do you want me to call them now so they know what's happening?' He's a little mocking but trying his best to help.

'Don't be ridiculous. That'll look ridiculous.' I'm laughing but I want to look less crazy so I tell him about my healing hands and the heat that I felt coming from them. He reaches out to touch them but they're clammy now.

'They're freezing cold.'

I deflate, wondering if I'm deluded.

Oscar's out like a light. He never has any trouble sleeping. I'm lying in the bed next to him, with the sheet over my head, tent-like, my knees propping it up. It's like we're in a coffin. A beautiful white double-sized coffin. I wonder who I will be buried next to. If I'm to spend eternity in the ground then it matters who's beside me, and I feel a sudden panic to know who that would be.

'Hello,' I hear from the silent and sleeping Oscar.

'Hello,' I hear me telepathically respond. Hearing Oscar's thoughts doesn't trouble me. It feels natural and right and reassuring. Perhaps we'll be buried together.

I can't get to sleep so I sit up, wrapping my arms around my knees. My body feels light as a feather. Hunched over, my arms are like a fledgling stuck in the nest for too long, all scrunched up. I stretch them out, like wings, flapping them a little, getting ready to fly.

'What are you doing?' Oscar's woken up.

'Just having a stretch. I can't sleep. Go back to sleep.'

In the morning, Oscar goes to work saying he'll call me later to see how I am. I stay in bed even though I'm not sleeping. A crowd of friends joins me but I'm pretty sure Oscar wouldn't be able to see them. I can't either but I can understand what they're saying. They seem like they're somewhere just above my head.

'I'm so excited. I remember when this happened to me.'

'Me too.'

'It's such a precious moment.'

They're not exactly voices because I can't hear them like I heard Oscar's voice in my head. They're more like blocks of thought coming into my brain like an email pinging into an inbox. Somehow my mind, like software, opens the message and it spills out with a character all of its own.

'Welcome. Welcome.'

There must be at least five of them, a team of spirits, who seem to have been assigned to me. They are excited by my sudden ability to 'hear' them.

'What's happening?' I ask none of them in particular and all of them at once.

'We're celebrating your union.'

'My union? So where's my big white dress?' I say, assuming that a union is a wedding.

'You're wearing a white dressing gown aren't you?' they respond, amused.

'So what about my wedding present?' I ask, joining in the fun.

'Over there by the radiator. The package on the floor. That thing you got the other day from the garage.' On the floor is a box containing a hands-free mobile phone kit for the car. A cameraman bought it for me on our way back from a recent shoot filming the Princess of Norway. They were on offer with fuel purchases and he thought five pounds was a bargain. So much so that when he asked me if I wanted one too, I was caught up in his enthusiasm, and said yes even though I'll prob-ably never use it.

'The hands-free kit? Sorry, I already opened it.'

'No one can resist opening a present.' They laugh.

A hands-free kit. It makes sense. I'm learning to communicate with-out hands, without a mobile, telepathically. I get it. They're playing with me. Teaching me to let go of the trappings of wedding dresses, gadgets, and phones.

'So what do we do now? You're not going to make me run down the street naked are you?' I ask, worried they'll deliberately try to make me look like a stereotypical crazy person.

'Only if you want to!' They're joking with me again but at the same time it's a serious reminder that I don't have to do anything I don't want to do. Apparently, they're not *those* kind of voices.

I'm told that we can all hear each other's thoughts now so we have to be quieter and respect each other's peace. I tiptoe across the room to the chest of drawers, trying to make as little noise as possible. Opening the drawers without making a sound is difficult. The wood squeaks and doing it slowly only prolongs it. I'm never going to get the hang of this; I'm sure my noisy clatter is disturbing everyone.

Then I hear Oscar's thoughts through the airwaves, even though he's a couple of miles away at his desk.

'I'm trying to work!' he pipes up. 'Keep the noise down.'

Oh dear, he's in on it too.

A split second later, the phone rings. It's Oscar calling to check if I'm OK.

'I'm fine.' I don't really know what else to say. I'm a little stunned he's called in the precise moment he's telepathically talking to me. I realise he probably has no idea that he's just psychically communicated with me and I'm stuck for words.

Once we hang up I wonder about the ramifications of this sudden new psychic ability. It's clearly disturbing Oscar's work so we'll have to take shifts to be awake. Oscar will get the day shift and go to work whilst I sleep. Then, when Oscar goes to bed, I'll stay awake. It means we'll never get to see each other, which is kind of tragic. I shouldn't complain, though, because we'll always be connected. I may have lost the daytime but I will have gained a whole network of psychic friends instead.

The front door opens but it doesn't sound like my lodger. I head down the stairs meeting Oscar on the tiny landing halfway. We hug and my body melts into his, meeting somewhere beyond our flesh, sharing an exquisite kiss, which I disappear into, like diving into a warm sea.

My legs give way as my body breaks down in tears. I drop onto the floor sobbing, but I know nothing of this because I'm somewhere else, in the imaginary kiss. At a loss as to what to do, Oscar drags me back up the stairs to my room. I've blacked out.

Once I come round, Oscar and my old housemate, Jess, are sitting in the front of the car whilst I'm in the back. In their awkwardness they are behaving like teenagers, talking about music and flicking the buttons on the stereo. I feel completely ignored. Jealousy creeps in to make sense of their giddy behaviour. Maybe they're secretly seeing each other. I'm not with Oscar any more and it would be hard to see him with somebody else, especially a good friend.

They take me to the GP who wants to put me in hospital but Oscar and Jess don't want that. I don't seem to be getting any say. The conversation is taking place without me and I'm being referred to in the third person.

'We'll keep an eye on her,' Jess says.

'We'll contact her parents,' Oscar adds.

Back home, I lie on the sofa and Jess pulls a chair up close and holds my hand. She strokes it gently. I look into her face and she smiles warmly. Her large eyelids give her a relaxed droopy-eyed look and her thin, top lip reveals her cute, ever-so-slightly rabbit-like teeth.

The quantum particles that make up her features rearrange themselves. A different version of her shines through like a long-lost friend from a past life. She's a girl in a wheelchair with wonky eyes. I see into the beauty of her soul, tender and kind, soft and loving.

'You are *so* beautiful,' I tell her.

She smiles back, her eyes filling with tears.

My elder brother, Sol, turns up relieving Oscar and Jess of their carer roles. My parents arrive a little later, having interrupted their holiday in Scotland. Sol cooks dinner; some kind of stir fry with baby sweet corn that looks like it came out of a science lab. I don't know when I last ate so I shovel it down.

'How's the food?' he asks. He's normally quite a good cook.

'It tastes like shit.'

Sol laughs, but I'm not joking. It reminds me of rotting cabbage.

When it's time for bed, I can't sleep again. My parents and brother are downstairs drinking Old Speckled Hen and chatting noisily. I look around my bedroom, taking in each object and picture. My eyes rest on a photo of the Twin Towers that I took on a trip to New York. The picture is taken from Brooklyn Bridge at night and the criss-crossing of the wire suspension in the foreground is out of focus. Orange lights shine from every window, like the souls of those lost in the catastrophe. Moved by the beauty of it, tears roll down my cheeks as I remember the events nearly eighteen months ago on September 11, 2001.

I was working in Norwich at the time, sitting with my editor, cutting together an eight-hour show presented by Michaela Strachan for *Animal Planet*. Watching the second plane fly into one of the buildings was surreal. It was like watching a movie. I had to remind myself it was actually happening live on the news.

Now, I think of the perfect part that everyone played in the epic drama of that day. Even the terrorists, though I'll never condone their actions, believed they were doing good. I feel a connection with the whole of life, in all its apparent imperfections. Right and wrong forming a paradox, like a bomb blowing apart all thinking and opening up a channel to my heart. A love fills me, rushing through my sobbing chest, adding sweetness to the tears. An unconditional love, even for the terrorists, cleanses me, washing away all fear, all blame, all cynicism, and all negativity.

* * *

Dad waits for me at the front door. I think we're heading up north again, back to my parents' house. Mum's already in the car. As I reach the bottom of the stairs a strange and uncomfortable sensation cripples me, taking me to my knees. It's hot and prickly and nauseating but not like I'm going to be sick. I just feel like a very, very bad person. Dad takes my hand and leads me out.

The reason for the journey has not been made explicit. Perhaps it's obvious to them but I'm confused. Maybe they're taking me to my wedding. They must be. A secret wedding that's been arranged to celebrate my union.

I have a recurring dream about a wedding. In it, my family and friends are secretly arranging my betrothal but I'm not supposed to know about it. I play along, feigning ignorance but desperate to know who my husband is going to be. It's incredibly frustrating and deceitful and I never make it to the altar. No one in the car is talking. It feels more like a funeral. Mum is heavy with emotion and Dad is concentrating on the road. All the cars are going at the same pace alongside us. The traffic on the other side of the motorway has piled up. Not a single car is moving. They're stuck in the end-of-the-world-traffic-jam-fuck-up that I suspect I'm the cause of, the tailback to my funeral.

CHAPTER SEVEN

Infinity

My parents' living room is crowded with my sister, her husband, and their son, as well as my mum and dad, all watching the TV. I don't know what they're glued to on the box. I'm not aware of the space around me. Perhaps I've closed my eyes—it seems dark and I've fallen down into the underworld or something. I don't really know. I'm not really focused so much on *where* I am as *who* I am.

I'm an old witch who speaks through gestures and actions, all that she's been through. I roll onto the floor, arching my back, with the top of my head touching the carpet. As I rotate it around, feeling the first vertebra twist on its axis, I know that once upon a time this old witch had her neck broken. Perhaps she was hanged. Maybe it was just me in a past life.

There are four of us now: me, my housemate Pippa, Kylie Minogue, and a fourth girl I'm not clear about. We're the cornerstones of a master plan, each holding court in our allocated corner of the globe, where we've been carefully placed. Like the shadowy silhouettes from the title sequence of the 1970s cult series *Charlie's Angels*, glamorous women armed and dangerous. We're gonna shoot the shit out of you, the KKK, Kylies Karrying Kalashnikovs. You better watch out 'cos these witch bitches are coming!

Nobody in the room says anything or tries to stop me. I can't stop myself either. I'm living a strange tale that wants to be told—the ultimate in body language.

I get up off the floor and now I'm on a horse. We're galloping along a track, the horse has bolted and I'm terrified. I lose my stirrup and let myself fall off. Then I'm climbing a rock, falling back down to the ground. Now I'm up again, pedalling across the room on a bicycle. I get knocked off by a car door opening in front of me. I get up once more and walk across the road and am hit by an oncoming bicycle. I get back on my bike and am hit by another vehicle, throwing me over the handlebars and onto the bonnet.

All of this I do in slightly slow motion, aware that these are all the ways I myself have come close to death. Every action is a re-enactment of an accident I've had. When it's finished, I pick myself up, brush myself off, and sit back in the chair.

What the fuck was all that about?

* * *

There's not much floor space in my bedroom, just enough to lie down on. It's the room I grew up in, aged eight to thirteen, and I sleep well in here. I used to have my rosettes on the wall and a picture of me riding my pony, Teacake. It was a great shot of us in the beginners' jumping. We're halfway over a jump, and I'm looking ahead to the next fence while Teacake is clearing the jump effortlessly, eager to please.

It was the summer before we moved to Hong Kong and I had saved up all the money I could get my hands on to pay the entry fees to my local shows. I squirrelled away my school dinner money, rather than wasting precious resources on a cooked meal. Instead, I scrounged two pence change off people in the ice cream van queue, which, added together, paid for a packet of crisps and a Nobbly Bobbly. I was determined to win the beginners' jumping before we left England. I'd entered it a few times but always got beaten. You didn't actually have to be a beginner: as long as you hadn't won it before you qualified. This show, just before our departure to the Far East, was my last chance and I had my heart set on that trophy. The photo captures my single-minded focus and unwavering concentration. The satisfaction I got from winning was equal to, and reflected by, the efforts I had put in.

The wallpaper, curtains, and furniture are all different now but the familiar shape of the room hasn't changed and it's comforting.

Sometimes when I'm stressed out about money and work, when shopping and cooking for myself feels like a huge effort, I want to come back home and be financially supported and have all my meals cooked for me. My parents have managed to provide that kind of secure, stable environment, despite the constant moving around the world.

I scan the bookshelf and a small lilac Bible jumps out at me. It's a soft leather-bound one, quite old. Mum is not religious. She's only kept it for sentimental reasons. Her brother and sister-in-law gave it to her when she was their bridesmaid. I pick it out, sliding it gently away from its neighbours. Placing it in the middle of the floor, I lie down on it, nestling it between my shoulder blades.

The book pushes against a place in my spine that feels like it wants to crack, like something lodged in my back wants to be set free. I let out an 'ah' sound and it feels good.

'Ahhhhh.' It gets louder and the louder it gets the better it feels. Then, opening my mouth wider, I make even more noise.

'AHHHHHHHHHHHHHHHHHHHHH.'

I'm lying with my arms out to the sides, like a crucifixion. Thinking about Jesus fuels my scream, a perfectly controlled note from a single breath, which gradually turns to anger. I'm mad about Christ being nailed to a cross, about killing a messenger of love and forgiveness. I can't comprehend why anyone would want to do that.

The sound fills the quiet house and Mum rushes upstairs.

'What's going on? What's wrong?' She opens the door to find me on the floor. I stop screaming and stand up revealing the Bible. I can't explain myself and don't even try. Mum bends down and picks up the book.

'What are you doing with that?' She snaps. I don't know what to say. She stuffs it back in its place.

'Fucking Bible,' she mutters.

Something else to blame religion for.

* * *

Every night Mum and I go through the same routine. She brings me the antipsychotic medication and gets worked up to make sure I take it. To her, it's a simple chemical problem with a simple chemical solution: too much dopamine. Antipsychotics prevent the uptake of dopamine in the brain's receptors. *Voilà*. All fixed. Having completed the first year of a nursing course, twice, and worked for years as a GP receptionist, she holds much faith in our medical system. To me it's a chemical lobotomy.

'Here, take this,' she says holding out two tablets in the palm of her hand. Every night I go through the same questions.

'What are they?'

'They're pills to make you better.'

'But what are they?'

'A blue pill and a white pill.' This is like *The Matrix.*

'But what do they do?'

'They make you better.'

'Better than what?'

'They make you well. Please take them.'

'I don't want to take them.'

'Please.' She sounds desperate.

'How will they make me well?'

'I don't know. Just take them.'

'You believe these will make me better?'

'Yes, so would you please just take them?' She sounds quite frustrated, like she gets when toddlers won't do as they're told.

So I take them.

For her.

Mum has read all about brain chemical imbalances, serotonin and dopamine theories, which have become popular knowledge since I first learned about them in psychology ten years ago. What isn't yet common knowledge though, is the work of award-winning medical journalist, Robert Whitaker, and his book *Mad in America*, published in 2002. Robert was horrified to learn that a person's chance of recovery from psychosis is much higher in developing countries like India or Nigeria than so-called developed countries like the US or UK. When he looked into it he found that, in spite of over 100 years of research and many billions spent, there was still no clear evidence that schizophrenia and other related psychotic disorders were the result of a diseased brain.

He uncovered shocking historical records that outlined how the public was sold a lie in order to sell more drugs. The drug companies had invented a story about a brain chemical imbalance to explain why antipsychotic medication worked. In fact Clozapine, the first antipsychotic developed in the 1950s, had only been shown to sedate patients making them less bothered by their symptoms. Psychiatrists at the time never reported cures, just that patients were easier to manage. The pharmaceutical industry has been running quite a racket and paying

psychiatrists to write articles for journals on the miracle cure of antipsychotics and Robert Whitaker's book exposes this.

For me, the drugs add another layer to the altered state I'm already
struggling to deal with.

I turn the light out and pull the covers over me, the medication making its way into my system. A blood red, hot liquid snake swallows my
feet, inching its way up my legs to my waist. There are holes at the tips
of my toes and something is draining out of me, taking with it all tension. My groin is being pulled downwards as the snake has me in its
mouth. My mouth joins in. Silvery saliva pools on my tongue, which I
press to the roof of my pallet. It spills into my throat so I swallow. My
eyes fill with a salty sting, blood like.

I've become the snake.

* * *

I wake to the sound of a text coming in. I've forgotten to turn my phone
off. There's hardly any signal at my parents' house but I can just about
get texts if I lean my mobile on the window ledge. I'm so sensitive, I can
feel the crap it's emitting, a crackling toxic buzzing that others seem
numb to. I reach up to check who the message is from. 'Oscar Mob'. My
inbox is full of texts from people's mobs, as if every individual comes
as a gang. I hadn't noticed this double meaning before. I don't want
gangster friends. I scroll though my contacts: Pippa Mob, Jane Mob,
Jess Mob, all new friends since my last episode. I've managed to rein-
vent my life but there's still something not quite right. I'm becoming
spiritual and my media friends are not really into that kind of thing. In
fact, they would probably mock it. Oscar did. I ponder the loss of my
relationship with him, which is still difficult even though it's been a
while since we split. It's hard to leave someone you love.

I need some spiritual friends: people who are open to possibilities
and won't take the piss out of me for it. What if I do have healing hands?
I imagine myself as a healer, piously doing everything perfectly right.

The word 'Pope' flashes up on the screen of my mobile, just long
enough for me to read it. It's not a text message from anyone. It simply
appears for a second and is gone again. Pope? My network of psychic
friends is teasing me again.

Who do I think I am?

I smile. I love their sense of humour. They're so irreverent.

I check Oscar's text. He's just asking how I am. 'Okay, OK.' I reply before deleting his message. I'm not repeating myself for effect. His initials are OK.

* * *

A social worker visits to see how I'm doing. He's wearing drab, uniformly dark colours that wash out his already winter-paled face, highlighting the dark rings under his eyes. He asks the usual question, common to all mental health staff.

'How are you doing?' It's not a very useful question. Taken literally, it requires a judgement of my actions so I ignore it.

'Er … you're all in black and don't look too well to me.' I'm sure he's going to be offended by my honesty but instead he smiles, genuinely amused. I've forgotten insults pass for humour up north.

'You seem better.'

'Really?'

'Yeah. Last time I came to call you wouldn't see me.'

'Oh. I don't remember that.' I can't even recall his visit.

'Exactly. So you've made progress. Do you mind if I stay and chat for a while?'

Chat is a euphemism for 'go through a relapse avoidance therapy pack'. Now that it's happened twice, it might be helpful to see if I can recognise the early warning signs. He has some cue cards with words that describe feelings, sensations, and thoughts that I might have had in the weeks leading up to my episode. If I could detect these early on then I might be able to avoid a full-blown psychosis in the future.

They're laminated A4 cards, black background with large white letters printed on them. Whoever designed them had no idea about the effects of colour. Already I'm put off, the blackness pressing some kind of evil alert button inside me.

'I'm going to hold each one up and you tell me whether you recognise it as an early symptom. OK?'

'OK.' He holds up the first card.

Suicidal.

'No.'

Thoughts of the devil.

'No.'

Paranoia.

'No.'

Receiving personal messages from the TV or radio.

'No.'

Hearing voices.

'No.'

If these are early warning signs I pity the poor fucker's full-blown psychosis. I'm irritated and feel patronised. This is for kids, holding up cards with words on.

'None of these are relevant,' I tell him.

'Well, how about you tell me what you experienced leading up to it?'

'There wasn't any warning.'

'There's usually something. Think about the days and weeks before and what was going on.' I rack my brains to remember anything odd.

'I remember a couple of days before knowing who was going to be next in the chair on *Who Wants to Be a Millionaire*.'

'Well, that's a start. Let's write it down and see what else we can find.' I like his adaptability, but I'm suspicious. Does he think this precognition was an early warning sign? Perhaps he sees psychic abilities as a symptom. I close up and decide not to tell him about my healing hands. I know how that will be perceived.

* * *

Out of curiosity, and because I've got a lot of time on my hands, I rummage around the attic to see what old stuff of mine is up there. There's a box of letters and cards that go back to when I was a teenager. I dust it off and carry it down the loft ladder.

When our family moved to Hong Kong, when I was thirteen, I wrote to all my friends. They all wrote back, taking much longer to reply than I did. I thought it meant they didn't care as much as me. Now I know I'm just more motivated like that.

An old Rag Mag jumps out at me. Every kid I hung out with in the village has written something silly and signed their names all over it. I read each entry, their different characters leaping from the page. And then I notice it's a Keele University Rag Mag. I had no idea back then that Keele would be the university I would go to.

I'm suddenly moved by the perfection of my life and flooded with a love for myself. A well of grief opens up and swallows me whole. I cry for ever thinking they didn't love me. I cry for missing them all so much. I cry all the tears I never cried back then because I didn't understand what

I was going through. I cry for all the people I've since lost touch with, and all the ways I imagine that people don't love me. There is so much love in this little box of letters and cards that I wonder how I never saw it before.

* * *

Mum shows her love through worry and food. She cooks proper, wholesome meals every evening. From scratch she makes shepherd's pies, fish pies, authentic curries, roast dinners, Bolognese, real chips, Yorkshire pudding. The list goes on. Often she pulls a recipe book from the shelf, usually by the latest celebrity chef, and follows it to the letter. When she places the food on the table she always apologises for something, as if her home-made efforts are inferior.

One evening, just as she's saying sorry for serving parsnips with fish, I pick up my knife and fork ready to tuck in. I pause, cutlery in hand, feeling a buzzing, like something's flowing in the metal. An invisible current is moving in gentle, continuous waves.

'Can anyone else feel something in the metal?'

'No. There's nothing in the knives and forks, Emma.' Dad is trying to reassure me but I don't like his implying I'm imagining it just because he can't sense it. Metal conducts energy. It's not so far-fetched. I focus on eating, carefully directing the peas and mash onto my fork with the knife and lifting it up to my mouth, trying not to let it distract me. Mum gets up from the table and reaches for some plastic camping cutlery from the dresser.

'Here. Use these,' she says, placing them by my plate.

'Thanks, Mum.'

It's only Mum, Dad, and myself in the house and we're all very quiet, the quietness of people who've lived together for a long time. It's comfortable and natural.

A silver flash catches my attention from the corner of my eye. I decide to ignore it. If I'm hallucinating, I'm not going to get drawn in. But there's another one and another one and every split second or so they're lighting up across the room. I'm not hallucinating. I'm going to figure this out. I pick them out and notice they're all coming from the direction of the windows. They must be coming from outside. *Maybe it's fairies in the garden.* I entertain myself with that thought. I don't believe in stuff like that, but I'm not ruling it out. There's hopefully some other, less wacky explanation.

Mum never closes the curtains in the evening so the windowpanes are blackened by the night, making them reflective. Spreading my attention wider, I see it: a brief flash as Dad lifts his fork up to his mouth, and then another as he moves his knife. It's just a reflection.

Phew. Mystery solved.

* * *

I move into Solomon's old bedroom, which is more spacious and overlooks the back garden instead of the road. I like the exposed, wooden floors, and the furniture doesn't take up all the space in the room like mine does. Lying in bed, with sparrows chirping in the hedges, readying themselves for the first of this year's clutch, is peaceful. The back of the house overlooks an old stone barn with resident little owls. Beyond are hilly fields with a crystal clear stream and well-tended sheep. It's a good place to convalesce.

My senses are dulled again, and the world is back to what is considered normal. But I feel sad. I miss it. I liked finding the network of psychic beings assigned to me. I liked feeling the magic of life. I want it back. In the corner of the room a shining point of light appears, a foot or two away from the walls. It moves quickly tracing a sideways figure of eight shape, like a child might outline a butterfly with a sparkler: the infinity sign. There isn't any trick of the light, no mirrors. I'm not hallucinating, though I'm sure my parents wouldn't be able to see it. I absolutely know for sure that it is as real as the birds outside. Not physical, but still real all the same. Some kind of light is pulsing into this realm so that I see it. I don't know what it is. I don't think to ask. The message it brings is one of hope. Like it's saying, 'Hey you, the magic *is* real.' I don't tell anyone about it though. Their reaction would only weaken my resolve.

CHAPTER EIGHT

Shiatsu

I don't hang around too long at my parents' house this time. I'm keen to get back to Bristol because I've signed up for an introductory shiatsu course. I'm intrigued by this mysterious Japanese practice and it might be a good way to sort myself out. I'm hoping to find out why I become psychotic.

It's not the first time I've tried to learn shiatsu. I found an evening class soon after my first episode but the week it started I broke my hand when a car door opened in front of me across a cycle lane. I couldn't do it with my wrist in plaster, so I gave my place to Nicky, the friend who I thought needed it most. I met Nicky through Ella. They were at uni together and we became friends immediately. Nicky has adopted a posture that says '*I don't really care*', but I know it's just a cover-up. I bumped into her a while back, and when she mentioned being in the first year of a professional practitioner training course, I was quite jealous. That was supposed to be me. I'd forgotten all about shiatsu and without a second thought I signed up to an introductory course at the same school.

We start by pairing up and spending five minutes each introducing ourselves. I'm sitting next to one of the assistants, Sean, so partnering with him seems obvious. He's only just finished the three-year course and loved it so much he wants to do it all again as an assistant. When he talks about the residential that happens at the end of the third year he becomes quite animated.

'Ken is an amazing man.'

'Who's Ken?' I ask.

'Ken Roberts. He's the principal of the school.' I don't know anything about the school. Nicky did the research to find it and I just went on faith that it must be the best one.

We ease into the course with some fun exercises. I pair up with a girl who blindfolds me and spins me around. With only verbal instructions she has to guide me to a chair and have me sit in it. It's obviously a trust exercise to break the ice.

'Turn to your right a little. OK. Now walk forwards a few paces.' I take a tentative step and it feels like I'm going to walk off the edge of a cliff.

'Stop. Side step to your left. *Good*. Take a step backwards.' Moving sideways and backwards feels fine but I don't understand why going forwards is so scary.

We circle up afterwards and the teacher, Jill, asks us all how we got on. I tell the group about how different it felt walking forwards, as opposed to sideways or backwards.

'You feel like you're going to walk off a cliff.'

'I,' Jill says.

'What?'

'You mean "I".'

'I feel like I'm going to walk off a cliff,' I correct myself. Saying 'I' instead of 'you' makes me feel quite exposed and vulnerable.

'That's your earth,' Jill says.

'My earth?'

'It indicates an imbalance in the earth element. You'll learn more about it on the course.' I've no idea what she means but I'm in, so I sign up for the first year.

* * *

I've qualified for a free trip to Europe with some points I've been collecting so I invite a few people to come with me to Prague. Only Oscar is interested so it's just going to be the two of us. Maybe it's what I secretly wanted. Even though we're not together, I still love him and am finding it hard to move on.

I don't really listen to the travel rep properly when I call to make the booking. She says something about my first choice not being available but her words don't fully register. I just say yes to everything she says. When she tells me how close to St Marks Square the hotel is, a linear train of thought connects Prague with communism and Karl Marx. St Marx Square. It makes total sense. But something feels off.

When the tickets arrive, they are two return flights to Venice. I'm embarrassed explaining this to Oscar, but he's amused by my cock-up. I don't often make mistakes and it probably levels the playing field. I just think it's ironic that we're going to the most romantic city in the world.

* * *

As part of the shiatsu course requirements, we have to have at least six treatments from a Shiatsu Society qualified practitioner in our first year. I book mine in with the founder and principal of the school, Ken Roberts. Ken has a prominent nose and thinning hair and a large crease, just like mine, between his eyes. He's not like anyone I've ever met. He's so full of life that I can't actually tell how old he is. He's definitely much older than me but he could be fifty or sixty or anywhere in-between.

I wait in reception, a little nervous until Ken comes for me and leads me to his treatment space. The room is minimal with only the necessary items: a futon mattress, a couple of chairs, and a box of tissues. I tell him briefly about my episodes and I get quite lively describing the questions I was asked in my first admission. His facial responses indicate empathy and amusement.

'Wow. What a journey you've been on,' he declares sincerely. His acknowledgement goes a long way and somewhere deep down inside I feel seen and loved. I'm not used to this kind of attention.

'Have you read *Women Who Run With the Wolves* by Clarissa Pinkola Estés?'

I shake my head.

'I highly recommend it. The introduction really struck me. Sometimes I reread that bit because there's so much in it.'

Ken stands up, takes his shoes off, and makes a gesture for me to lie on the mat.

He hones in on sore places that feel bruised, occasionally pausing to scratch his nose. He reaches under my neck and cups my head. Holding me gently and firmly, it's easy to rest the heavy weight of my head in his hands. He moves it slowly, rotating left and right slightly, with his fingers probing the bones in my neck. With a sudden jolt he slams my head fully right and I hear a massive crack that reverberates through my whole body like a large gong being struck sending a shock wave through my system. My heart is pounding, heat rises through my face, and I have one thought and one thought only.

Get out! Get the fuck out!

I mentally map where the door is, behind me and to the right but I lie still, containing the earthquake that's erupting inside me. It's just a panic attack. I've had a few before. I trust this man. He knows what he's doing.

Ken lowers his hands resting them beneath my head and doesn't move for what seems like ages. I don't know if he can tell what's happening to me.

Is he waiting for me or is this pause part of the treatment? More heat flushes through my face. I'm embarrassed that I'm taking so long to settle. The uncomfortable squirming and fear eventually subside.

When the session is finished I make sure I don't leave without getting the details of the book.

'Can you write the name down of that author for me? I'll never remember it.'

'Sure,' he says reaching for his notebook. 'Clarissa Pinkola Estés.' He hands me the piece of paper and I put my shoes on, thanking him profusely. The assistant was right. Ken Roberts is an amazing man.

Back home I feel great. I put on a Nitin Sawhney album and stand in the middle of the room listening to the evocative sounds of the Indian instruments. A weird banjo-like thing slides into a bluesy guitar. Then a male voice hums alongside a contemporary beat. A high female vocal in Hindi joins in, followed by a distant New York rapper. I love the way Nitin fuses contemporary with traditional Asian instruments.

I grab the plastic handle of a synthetic white feather duster, and dance. Standing with my feet shoulder-width apart, my hips pulse to the beat. The first song is all about a river flowing deep inside. There's a strange pull in my lower belly, like a trickling stream: the river flowing through me. I raise my right arm up to reach the cobwebbed corner above the stereo. A silky, liquid, golden ribbon of light flows from the handle to just below my belly button, where it is anchored. As I move the duster upwards, the ribbon grows longer, instead of breaking, as if its length is infinite. The gold looks multicoloured, reflecting pink, purple, and orange, like oil does on water. It looks like CGI from a movie. I move my hand back towards me and graceful folds take up the slack of the excess ribbon. It's the most beautiful thing I've ever seen. They are perfectly spaced, sized, and curved, the way a real silken ribbon would curl and bounce, if it didn't completely succumb to gravity.

I dance on through to the kitchen. My body feels light and agile, a magical ribbon dancer.

What if I'm hallucinating?

A jolt of fear freezes me. And then the ribbon is gone.

* * *

I treat myself to the book Ken mentioned, *Women Who Run With the Wolves* and devour the introduction.

'I'll tell you right now, the doors to the world of the wild Self are few but precious. If you have a deep scar, that is a door, if you have an old, old story, that is a door. If you love the sky and the water so much you almost cannot bear it, that is a door. If you yearn for a deeper life, a full life, a sane life, that is a door.

How did Ken know I needed to read this book? It makes my psychosis seem like a doorway to something bigger: my wild and true Self.

* * *

We sit *al fresco* to enjoy Italian coffee near the busy Piazza San Marco: 'St Marx Square'. I soak up the autumn sun and watch the world of Venice go by. Since the shiatsu treatment, I've felt quite serene and I don't feel overly chatty. Oscar and I are comfortable with our silence.

A small boy pulls along his favourite wooden truck with string. I know it's his favourite because he looks so pleased with himself. He loves this truck like it's a dog on a lead. An orange aura, like the Ready Brek advert in the Eighties, surrounds him and stretches backwards, wrapping around the little wooden vehicle, like the toy and the boy are one thing. I didn't know auras did that. Oscar is watching me watch the boy and it reassures me.

The child speeds up to catch up with his mother, his little lorry an extension of himself. He looks back over his shoulder to check the truck is still there, and disappears around the corner.

We've booked tickets to see a string quartet performing Vivaldi's *Four Seasons*, which isn't the kind of thing either of us would normally go to but it's so cultured in Venice that a classical concert feels compulsory. It's one we both know. Who doesn't?

It's a fairly small space, and the audience is sitting at the same level as the musicians. As the music begins, I try to picture a spring landscape so that I can connect with what Vivaldi was trying to portray. But it's no use. I'm distracted, searching for the advert I'm only half remembering. Maybe it's an airline company. Marco Polo Business Class with Cathay Pacific? Definitely something trying to get across a sense of class. I lure myself away from this thought by deliberately imagining a fawn frolicking in a woodland glade but that doesn't work either. It's usurped by an image of a bunch of people dancing around a Baroque ballroom in eighteenth-century grey wigs and too much white face powder. Then faint memories of another commercial steal my attention away again.

How am I supposed to enjoy this? The music has so many associations my ears are too biased to hear it properly.

Maybe I should stop trying so hard. Instead I focus on the musicians' bows moving in unison: two violins, a viola and a cello. I watch their fingers moving quickly across the strings and let out a sigh, relaxing into my seat.

Suddenly, around each player is a purple glow, the same colour I saw in the hospital seven years ago. When I tense up the auras disappear but when I relax they appear again. I deliberately tighten up and let go a few more times to check this theory. I can only see them when I'm in a relaxed state.

These auras are definitely not hallucinations.

Hallucinations are associated with a disturbed mind. They're visions that are considered not real because no one else can see them. Here, in Venice, I'm not at all disturbed. On the contrary, I'm consciously choosing to relax so I'm certain I'm experiencing a real phenomenon even though Oscar can't see it.

I know, too, that I saw the golden ribbon of light as a result of the shiatsu treatment. Somehow it activated a psychic visual sense, opened my third eye, perhaps. I definitely wasn't having an episode so maybe the auras I'd seen in my first psychosis weren't symptoms either. If I'm able to access weird stuff like this when I'm not psychotic, then maybe experiencing them during psychosis isn't a symptom of madness at all.

When I was doing my psychology degree, I took part in an experiment. I was curious about what the professors were researching, so I offered myself up as a subject. In this particular study I had to watch a series of images on a computer screen. In-between these pictures, a word would flash up, at a speed that was beyond my visual acuity.

This means that the words would appear and disappear so quickly that I wouldn't be able to consciously register seeing them. If I were asked if I'd seen anything, I would likely deny it, even though a word was being shown to me. I had to click makeshift buttons in my hands, made from old 35mm film canisters, to indicate whether I had seen anything or not: right hand for *yes*, left hand for *no*. I was told to let my hands decide, and allow them to answer of their own accord.

As I watched the images, not seeing a single word appear in-between them, I let my hands press away merrily. It was freaky, pushing the button for *yes* and the button for *no* without any real conscious command. It was as if my hands were connected to a different person, getting instructions from someone else. I wondered, as I so often did with psychology experiments, what they were really trying to measure. Was it a trick to see if I would do something silly because my professor, the head of the department, had told me to? Were they seeing how long I would do it before I objected? I bet they weren't really showing me any words at all! My hands were probably just clicking randomly. I felt stupid but I completed the task in spite of this.

At the end of my session, the professor checked the results and asked me if I could see any of the words. I assured him that I hadn't seen a single one. I didn't let on that I was actually feeling quite suspicious about the whole thing.

'Are you sure?' he asked. 'If you had got two more right, I would have had to increase the speed at which they were flashing on screen and repeat the experiment. The results suggest that you could see the words. Are you sure you didn't see anything?'

I was amazed that there was a part of me seeing things that the conscious me didn't know I was seeing. And not only that, my hands knew when I was seeing something even though *I* hadn't a clue. My perception was so keen that they nearly had to alter the experimental conditions because I was so far off the normal range expected.

Another interesting study—of which I was not a part—was conducted at Hannover Medical School in Germany, and University College London's Institute of Cognitive Neuroscience. It involved a hollow-mask experiment. Essentially, when we are shown a two-dimensional photograph of a white facemask, it looks exactly the same, whether it is pointing outwards, with the convex face towards the camera, or inwards, with the concave face towards the camera. It's known as the hollow-mask illusion. Such photographs were shown to a sample of

control volunteers. Sometimes the face pointed outwards, and sometimes inwards. Almost every time the hollow, inward-pointing concave
face was shown to them, they misrepresented it and reported that they
were seeing the outwards-pointing face of the mask instead. This mis-
categorisation occurred 99% of the time. The same experiment was then
performed on a sample of individuals with a diagnosis of schizophrenia.
They did not fall for the illusion. In fact, 93% of the time, this group was
actually correctly able to identify when the photo placed before them
was, in fact, an inward-pointing concave mask. This experiment suggests that, when it comes to visual perceptual ability, so-called normal
people are less in touch with reality than those with psychotic illness.

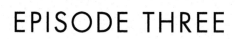

EPISODE THREE

CHAPTER NINE

Discovery

Shiatsu is a life changer. At my next shiatsu session with Ken, I tell him I feel nervous and jittery most of the time, butterflies in my stomach. He looks at me and pauses before asking,

'Are you open to the possibility of experiencing fear?'

'Yes,' I reply defensively, ruffled by the implication that I might not be.

'Nervous is just another way of saying fear,' Ken explains. I'm quiet as I think about it. Nervous is definitely lower on the scale, but I take his point. I'm shying away from using the word 'scared' because it makes me feel vulnerable.

'I think I may have been sexually abused as a child.' I don't know where the sentence comes from. It just pops out of my mouth, surprising me more than it fazes Ken.

'On one level, it doesn't matter,' he replies. I wonder on what level he means.

One of the other shiatsu teachers introduces us to something called qigong. It's a bit like tai chi. She recommends it because it can help us get in touch with chi, which is crucial for practising shiatsu. I'm in my second year of the course now and I still can't feel this strange energy force so I think I'd better go to the qigong class she plugs.

At the first class I feel intimidated. Everyone seems to know each other and they're all pally-pally, hugging each other in greeting. It's mostly men so I check out the room for the best-looking guy, even though that has nothing to do with why I'm here. I'm here to feel *chi*. If you can't feel *chi*, you can't really do shiatsu properly.

I feel a bit silly making weird movements and some people are making odd noises too. I'm not sure if they are just faking it, but I decide not to join them. We stand with our arms crossed at the wrists, eyes closed, feet shoulder-width apart, and knees off lock. The teacher, David, approaches me quietly. Even though my eyelids are shut, I can sense him watching me. My face flushes with the thought of what he must be thinking about me: how rubbish I am at it. He comes up close to me and makes the slightest, minuscule adjustment to my wrists. Immediately I feel my right wrist connect to my left at a central point, plugging into a circuit. This must be *chi*. How the fuck did he know to do that?

We stay like this for ages. I've no idea how long, maybe twenty minutes. I'm not really counting. I don't know what's meant to happen so I don't try to achieve anything. I just focus on feeling the weird buzzing in my wrists.

We change positions. This time, our arms are holding an imaginary ball of chi in front of us. I can feel something that might be chi, a kind of thick sea of air between my palms. My shoulders are aching so I breathe into the pain to release the tension causing the discomfort. They relax a little and the ache subsides before returning again for another release. We do this for another age.

'Emmm ... maaaaa ...' I hear my name being called from far away across the Downs, among the din of children playing. It lures me into a different state, one in which I've lost any sense of the physical boundary of my body. I'm as expansive as the entire cosmos. My consciousness is no longer located in my head. I'm everywhere. I feel euphoric, enjoying the out-of-body experience. Is this why people do qigong?

When we circle up at the end of the class, an opportunity to share, most people moan about the pain and the boredom. Some express their gratitude at the luxury of spending the whole day doing qigong. I want to tell them what an amazing time I've just had but worry they might get jealous and take a dislike to me so I keep quiet.

Learning to work with energy is confirming the existence of something I have experienced before. What I felt flowing through the knives and forks at the dinner table was *chi*, I just didn't know it then. It's ironic: I'm studying shiatsu to find out what's wrong with me, why I became psychotic, but I'm actually discovering there may be something very right with me.

* * *

My elder brother's moved to Spain. At the first opportunity I go and visit them, in the mountains in the north, near Alicante.

My sister's come too. Sally's older than me, by just under a year. I was born two days before her first birthday so effectively we're the same age for two days every year. She's very different from me, more materialistic and into make-up and glamour. She was always the one with the boyfriend, whilst I remained fiercely independent. I did better academically, but she has a secure and steady job with a pension. She travels a lot as cabin crew but stays in expensive hotels and dines in fancy restaurants. Whenever I go anywhere, I rough it in hostels with a backpack and sample the local street food.

I give Sally and my sister-in-law a shiatsu treatment because my course requires me to complete a certain number of them. They've never had it before and probably don't know what to expect.

After dinner Sally and my brother's wife, Gillian, remain sitting at the dining table finishing a bottle of red wine. Alcohol is not recommended after a shiatsu treatment as it interferes with the body's natural healing process. Because shiatsu can bring up buried emotions it's best not to cover them up with booze. I'm over on the sofa giving the vino a miss. Their kids have gone to bed, and they're both letting their hair down a little. I keep out of the conversation because it sounds like the wine is doing all the talking. I'm easily riled these days so prefer not to be there when the fight happens, if you know what I mean.

I think they're talking about paedophiles, in an anxious, *Daily Mail* kind of way. Not having a master plan for the conversation but wanting to bring up the subject with Sally, I butt in.

'I think I may have been sexually abused,' I say, unsure of myself.

'Didn't Mum tell you?' she responds, sounding surprised that Mum clearly didn't.

'No. She only told me you were.'

'We *both* were.'

She doesn't need to say it but hearing the words cuts through the shock and I bawl like a baby. Both of them move closer to sit beside me, but I'm inconsolable.

It all makes sense now: why I'm useless at relationships. I'm crying for the effect it's had on my adult life, one that I've been, until now, completely ignorant of.

'The *gardien* used to play with us on the patio,' Sally explains.

'I remember playing the bean game on the patio with the gardener.'

'No he wasn't a gardener. He was the *gardien*,' she corrects me.

'Oh. I thought we had a special bond.' Another penny drops. That's exactly what I heard another victim of sexual abuse say when I interviewed her for a documentary recently.

'You don't know it's wrong,' she said. 'Nobody goes around talking about it.'

As expats, we employed local people to help: someone in the kitchen and someone in the garden, keeping an eye on the house. The cook was caught stealing and got the sack but the guardian, or *gardien* in French, was supposed to ensure our security. I was only five or six.

My sister goes into some detail about what this man used to do to her and I'm not sure if she's trying to help or if misery seeks company. She probably just needs to offload. After all, she's kept it a secret all these years. It's not helping me, though, so I head off to bed where I can do all the crying I need.

Alone with my tears, memories come back to me.

Standing at the end of our neighbour's driveway with my knickers down, showing the boy down the road what I assumed he wanted to see. My sister looked horrified when she caught us, making it seem shameful. I wonder now whether it was healthy childhood exploratory behaviour I was engaged in, or something I had learned from the abuse.

I also remember being with my Mum at the house of a friend of hers, where they were having coffee. It was probably before I started school because my elder brother and sister weren't there; they would have been at school. I'm guessing I was four. I needed to go to the toilet but couldn't speak to ask where it was. I was so scared, I just didn't know what to say or do. I sat in a silent panic until I just peed right there, in the armchair I was sitting on. Perhaps this abuse is why I felt so afraid as a child. It might have set off a feeling of lack of safety within me that I had no way of expressing at that age.

I look at my nieces and nephews fast asleep, safely tucked up in bed. They're not much older than I was back then. I don't want to wake them so I stifle my sobs under the duvet.

* * *

My tutorial is at the principal's house. I've got to give him a short treatment and then he's going to tell me what my 'gift' is. I think calling it a 'gift' is just a way to make being judged seem more palatable. It doesn't make me feel any less nervous. I've also got something difficult to say to Ken, which is not helping my nerves.

'There's been a few times in class where I've felt shot down by you.'

'Oh …' He doesn't seem at all defensive so I go on to list a few incidents where I thought he was rather harsh in the way he corrected me in class. I don't need anything from him. I just need to learn to stick up for myself. Learning shiatsu is making me more aware of all the ways I've learnt to avoid stuff: emotions, conflict, and difficulty.

'I'm sorry,' he says. 'That's just my ego. I'll try to be more mindful in future.' His reply is so skilful I'm amazed, but also disappointed there's nothing for me to rail against. He's not very sympathetic sounding, though. Is he just dodging a bullet?

I continue with my next topic.

'I discovered recently that I was sexually abused. It brought up a lot of grief that I didn't know I was carrying. But you said that on one level, it didn't matter. I'm just wondering on what level it doesn't matter.'

'Did I say that? I don't remember.'

'Yes you did. And the thing is, I had a strange hunch and I needed to know. And it does matter. It makes sense of a lot of my life.' I'm aware that I'm in my thirties and my older siblings are married with children while my relationships don't last. Ken doesn't say anything, and I don't say any more about it either.

We move over to the mat to make a start. I'm really tense so I try to relax my arms. I've no idea what to do but I've been told he only wants to get a sense of the quality of my touch. I'm shaking and the last thing I want to do is put my hands on him: clammy, jittery, terrified hands. I take a deep breath and bravely get on with it.

At the end of the treatment, Ken sits up and smiles. He looks tired. He tells me that my touch invites surrender and trust. I'm not really listening because I no longer value his opinion. Instead I ask for help feeling *chi* in people. He demonstrates how to position yourself, with arms shoulder-width apart and soft at the elbows, his hands resting gently palms down on the mattress. As he's tuning in, he lifts his head and looks at me with surprise.

'I can feel the energy in the futon,' he says excitedly. 'I've never felt that before.'

I don't know what to say. I'm surprised this is the first time he's experienced this given how long he's been doing shiatsu. I've been feeling energy in objects since the qigong class. I felt it in the car seat on the way here. It's people I'm having trouble with.

'Wow, energy is in everything.' Ken is very animated by his new discovery. 'I could give my lawn a shiatsu and see if it grows any better. I could have a control sample patch to compare it to,' he laughs. I smile back enjoying the silly direction he's steered the conversation in. He's suddenly very childlike and has shrunk to a more human size.

'I've got a spare futon mattress that a second year student wants to pass on. They're not continuing with the course so they don't need it. Do you need one?' Ken asks. It feels a little bit like a gesture of apology, as he carries the heavy load out of his house and lifts it into the boot of my car.

CHAPTER TEN

Qigong

The qigong camp is in a field on the edge of Dartmoor, near Totnes. I've never seen such a bunch of raggle-taggle hippies: yurts, prayer flags, drums, compost loos, and women wearing skirts over their trousers. A couple from Yorkshire push their two chilled-out children around in a wheelbarrow. People hug each other for interminable lengths of time, swaying from side to side. It's not so much a greeting as an activity in itself. What a contrast with my trendy Bristol media friends.

We've been told to bring shampoo that's eco-friendly and bathe at least fifteen feet away from the stream so that Holy Brook, which flows into the River Dart, remains unpolluted by twenty-first century skin-care products. I pitch my cheap red nylon tent at the far end of the camping field, not quite part of it all, but not separate either.

There are so many welcoming induction sessions I wonder if it will ever get underway.

I make my way to the meditation tent and sit on a cushion. Barry, who runs the camp with my teacher, David, is leading this one. Barry and David both have receding hairlines but the similarity ends there. David is much darker skinned with an elegant Roman nose and thick pursed lips, like a Pre-Raphaelite painting. Barry looks like he may have had ginger hair at one time but it's faded now as they're both middle-aged. His thick-rimmed spectacles rest on his nose and his appearance is more rodent than Pre-Raphaelite. He introduces the guy sitting next to him as Michael. Michael is going to conduct the energies during the meditation, whatever that means. We're asked to close our eyes and focus inwards. I don't really know what I'm supposed to be doing. Sitting in silence soon gets boring so I open one eye to see what everyone else is doing. Michael's arms are flailing wildly like a traffic policemen gone mad. His face is being pulled in all directions contorting into expressions an animator couldn't make up. I'm fascinated. What the hell is he doing?

When the meditation is over, Barry opens up the circle for questions. *How do you meditate? What's meant to happen? What if it's really painful to sit cross-legged?* Michael answers them all. I think he's a little younger than Barry and David but he's obviously a pro at meditating, otherwise they wouldn't have handed it over to him to explain it all.

'When I first started meditating I thought I would be like those statues I've seen of the Buddha, peaceful and serene. Instead I got the urge to move my arms about and pull strange faces. It was hard to hold them back. I desperately wanted to be calm and still like everybody else but it was just easier to let my body do whatever it wanted to do.'

This guy is weird, but I like him.

I see him the next day sitting in a circle giving some kind of talk to a small crowd. He has messy blond hair and dark-rimmed glasses that make him look quite geeky. I'm really curious so I head over. As I approach I hear him say, 'I just want to love God.' What would have made me cringe a few years ago now sounds brave. It's such a simple and honest public declaration. How does he have the guts to say that in this day and age?

I sit down next to a woman who rearranges her pen and notebook. What has she brought those for? I'm baffled and amused by her studiousness. I don't think she'll find God there.

'There's a golden ribbon of light that comes out of the *dantien*, our centre, or power point just below the navel.' Michael describes a ribbon that connects from the light body to the physical realm. 'It attaches itself to whatever you're attached to, so imagine how horrified I was one day to discover that mine was connected to my TV.' Michael laughs at himself. My jaw drops. I couldn't find any mention of golden ribbons on the internet. So I'm not the only one who's experienced them. They *do* exist: this guy's seen them too!

* * *

Halfway through the ten-day camp, life has fallen into a healthy routine. I wake early and coax myself into the icy waters of Holy Brook for a morning cleanse. Sometimes I treat myself to the Heath Robinson hot shower. I rarely make it to the early qigong session but I'm always at the main class after breakfast. Afternoons are spent hanging out with my new friends by the River Dart or giving shiatsu treatments. Evenings range from meditation to sauna or dancing, to drumming or a singsong by the fire. I feel like I've been here forever.

On Wednesday evening there's a healing session in the main yurt. David, Barry, and Michael are running it and everyone is welcome, but nothing is compulsory. I want to see Michael at work. There are 100 people and I wonder how they're going to manage such a large group.

'We'll be working with the fire energy. There's nothing you have to do. The energy will go wherever it needs to go in your body,' Barry explains when he introduces it.

It sounds simple enough. We've been studying the Chinese system of five elements in shiatsu so I know about the fire: the energy of the heart, of love and it's what provides the alchemy for transformation. I've no idea how they'll isolate this energy and send it where it needs to go, though.

Barry, who is doing all the talking, guides us into a relaxed state. I watch David and Michael, curious to know what they're doing. Michael is manically moving his arms and face again. David looks more sedate, moving slowly and deliberately as if conducting an invisible orchestra. People are swaying around unpredictably, jerking this way and that. Some of them emit strange beast-like noises. I don't feel anything, and I can't help thinking they're all faking it to go along with the show. It's like they're hypnotised. Not having the urge to join them, I lie down on the ground and close my eyes.

The sound of horses' hooves galloping around in the next field tells me they're picking up something strange in the air and it's getting them all fired up. Suddenly, I'm aware that my upper body feels like it has tipped backwards below the earth, as if it's sloping downhill—but the ground is flat. It's like I'm hanging upside down. Perhaps it's just my energy body I'm tuning into.

'Gradually bring yourselves back into the space.' Barry is closing the session just as I'm finally relaxing into it. I'm not ready for it to be over yet. I'm only just getting started.

'If you want to stay and share your experience you're all very welcome.' I don't particularly want to sit around listening to the rest of the group so I get up and head out. I walk through the gate to the next field to say hello to the horses.

A beautiful chestnut gelding jolts his head up in the dark, snorting at me with flared nostrils. I approach him slowly, averting my gaze so as not to make direct eye contact. I also turn my shoulders at an angle, so they're not square on to him, to let him know I'm no threat. I learnt this from Monty Roberts, the original horse whisperer, who I met on a shoot for a series presented by the Princess of Norway.

Monty studied how horses communicate with each other by watching wild herds of mustangs. When a young colt is behaving antisocially, nipping or biting others, the matriach pushes him out. The worst thing that can happen to a herding animal is to be excluded, their safety being in numbers. Feeling vulnerable and exposed to predators, the youngster soon apologises. He does this by lowering his head and making a chewing action, which effectively means 'I'm ready to eat'. As soon as she sees this, the matriarch allows the young horse back in the herd and showers him with affection. Monty Roberts uses this method to train horses without using violence. He mimics the matriach by pushing the horse away until it apologises. He gets them to join up with him rather than break their spirits. Now he teaches the world how to use body language to make friends with your horse so that it willingly does what you ask, without the need for any force.

The gelding relaxes a little and sniffs my hand curiously. His whiskers tickle my palm and I lean forward to take in his scent. He smells of the wild, a delicious sweet smell of hay and oiled skin. His copper fur feels silky as I lightly stroke my hand along his solid neck. My senses seem sharper than usual.

Back in my tent I lie awake until the early hours of the morning. My belly is on fire, cooking me like a furnace from the inside. It's not unpleasant, just a heatwave burning through my body. This must be the fire energy. At around four o'clock I finally drop into a slumber.

I wake early with the sun glowing through my tent, lighting the inside of it pink. I'm clammy from night sweats but feel well, like a cleansing after an illness. Lying on my back, enjoying the freshness in the air, I'm not in any hurry to get up.

'Remember your union?' A disembodied thought, located somewhere above me, is talking to me again. I do remember it, my ridiculous dressing-gown wedding dress and hands-free kit present—which I was given after the shoot with Monty Roberts.

'Remember?'

It's not the crowd of spirits that came last time. This time there's only one and it feels like God, whatever *that* is. Apparently the union they were celebrating was with *Him*.

'But I want to marry a man and have children,' I say, turning away and rolling onto my front. I'm immediately aware of the futility of thinking I can turn away from something that is supposed to be omnipotent.

'You're to become a healer.'

'A healer?'

'There's nothing you need to do. People will come to you.' I'm flattered but not convinced. I like the idea of it, but it doesn't seem likely. Maybe it's something to do with my shiatsu.

A little concerned, I head over to the qigong field to catch David after the early morning session. David runs my class in Bristol and said he was really pleased I'd decided to join him for the camp. But he never asked for any emergency numbers or anything like that so I think it wise to let him know about my medical history. The early session has just finished but he's still busy in a conversation with Barry and Michael.

'Sometimes I like to give some people a little *chi* boost with my hands,' I overhear Barry boasting. David and Michael both nod in amused agreement. I wait until they finish their conversation and go their separate ways before I approach David.

'I need to tell you about my medical history,' I launch straight in. 'I have a history of psychosis, and I felt quite trippy after that healing session last night. I'm OK and there's probably nothing to worry about but just in case, I thought I'd better let you know.' If he's at all shocked, he doesn't let it show.

A hike on the moor is planned for the day, which I'm relieved about as it means there's no qigong. I don't think I need to do any more of it right now. I put on my walking boots and join the crowd up the bridle path and along the country lane towards Dartmoor.

I'm not feeling very social and I don't have anything to say so I walk alone among a convoy of chatting people. Once we're on the moor, we leave the road and head across the well-grazed land to Bench Tor, dropping into a pre-agreed silence. The Tor overlooks the River Dart, which disappears around a big bend in the distance. The valley down to it is covered in trees, mostly oak, which survived man's axe on this steep slope. Bench Tor is made up of a series of layered granite outcrops, exposed along the shoulder of the hill. They look like piles of giant cow-pats, having been formed by volcanic activity millions of years ago, the earth pushing up molten magma.

Lunch on the top takes place in a frenzy of excitement. Whipped up by the wind blowing on the exposed ridge, David is flitting around, in total contrast to his usual calm. A woman I don't really know attempts to have a conversation with me but I don't seem to have access to my usual social niceties.

Once we've all finished eating, we continue on down a path that enters the ancient woodland. The trees, stunted by the weather on the exposed hill are gnarled with age and dripping with moss. The ground is a vivid green with lichens and ferns covering large boulders wedged between the oaks. No wonder it has never been cut for grazing.

I stay silent while the others talk about trivial matters in which I have no interest, as we reach the bottom of the valley where the River Dart rages. Clothes are scattered along the bank. Some people are already swimming, naked, screaming and whooping with the cold. I peel off my T-shirt and navy blue corduroy trousers and tiptoe tentatively in. It tickles my calves and I wade in deeper, feeling the water hit my thighs. I count to three and dive in. It feels colder on certain parts of my body. A small patch on my upper back and a circle on the top of my head have no defence against the icy temperature. I get out quickly and wrap myself in a towel. The sensation in my middle fingers is beginning to go. They're turning yellow, like a dead man's fingers. Raynaud's. I put my palms on a large rock, heated by the sun, to warm them up. Something tugs like a magnetic force, plugging me into the rock.

We don't hang around long by the water, taking the path down-stream, through the woods. It's narrow and we all quickly spread out, going at our own pace. A patch of sun lights up a small clearing, and I'm drawn to stand in its centre. The heat of the sun warms me. I lift my head to the sky and close my eyes. Then I'm sobbing, and I've no idea why. I hear the low chatter of a few women approaching. They gather around, enfolding me in a circle. I let myself cry knowing that this kind of thing is welcomed on the camp. One of them puts her arm gently around my waist whilst another rests her head tenderly on my shoulder. Nobody speaks, and I'm comforted by the silence and their care.

Back at the camp people seem like caricatures, cartoon charac-ters of themselves. A woman in her forties is wearing a baseball cap backwards, cut off combats, and a pair of Nike trainers. They don't look right on her, too casual, too American, too teenage. Michael walks past muttering to himself.

'Tony Blair,' he says, under his breath, like a swear word but it doesn't make any sense so I wonder if I'm hearing things.

I zip up my tent to get away from the weirdness. But inside it's even more intense, a pink bubble with no air. I can't see what's going on outside and my ears are on hyper alert. The person in the next tent is scribbling profusely. I think she's writing my story. For posterity.

At dinner time someone shows up with a plate of food for me. They must have noticed I haven't come out of my tent for a while. Maybe David is keeping an eye on me.

* * *

I'm taken to see a doctor, but I don't remember leaving the camp. I vaguely recall freaking out in a car but I'm not sure if that just takes place in my head whilst I fake composure. I think we sit outside on the grass rather than go into the surgery itself. Some women from the camp are with me, feeding me apples or cakes or something that feels like a treat. It's all a bit of a blur.

A weird story about the GP forms in my head when he looks up from his computer and smiles at me. It's like he's been waiting for me for a very long time: a psychologist who's been studying me since uni and has figured out that I'm the reason they keep having to invent new drugs. As each new medicine loses its effectiveness, another must be created. They give it a name using the next letter of the alphabet as the first letter. I must have made my way through them all from Acid to Zopiclone. Now they've run out of letters, there's no more drugs to give me.

The GP must have told us to go to the hospital because the next thing I'm aware of is Barry driving me there. A woman in the passenger's seat is jabbering away to him like a long-lost pal. Once again, I'm not included in the conversation.

The waiting room is packed with people. Barry leans back with his hands clasped behind his head and an ankle crossed over his knee. It's an arrogant-looking posture, but his twitching foot gives away his nerves.

I must have blacked out again, because I wake to find myself in a bed in a small room but I don't remember how I got here, or even David arriving. He's sitting at the other end of the bed holding my gaze. I peer through my half-closed eyelids at him, silently keeping watch. A dark purple and green light is glowing around him.

It's unclear how I ended up in the ambulance but it's like being in an aeroplane cockpit with all the equipment and the switches and lights. I'm lying on one of those wheelie beds, narrow and plastic. A kind-looking woman is sitting next to me in a paramedic uniform. Her hands are gently laid in her lap and her head is tilted sympathetically towards me. I look back at her scrutinising the glow of light coming from her face. It's a similar purply green colour, shining from the contours of her features like a hologram. The image changes, fading into a different person's face. Every few seconds, a new visage appears.

Who are these people? They seem ancient and powerful, come to watch over me, to protect me. A woman who bears a resemblance to my sister's mother-in-law appears among the many other spirits. Maybe they're my ancestors, relatives from all the branches of my family tree, even the in-laws of my siblings.

CHAPTER ELEVEN

Sectioned

I'm shown around Dundry Villa, Barrow Gurney Hospital, which sounds like a haunted holiday camp in Ugly Town. It's so shabby: I feel like I'm here to inspect the place, expose it to the world. It's a mental institution built in the 1930s, progressive in its day but mostly boarded up now.

I'm given my own room on the main ward with a nurse stationed by my bed. I'm on twenty-four hour watch. Suicide watch, though I have no intention of killing myself, is standard procedure.

I drift in and out of a dreamlike state. God appears again but this time in human form, resembling David Attenborough. I'm inside one of those toy snow shakers and Sir David is rubbing his hands with total fascination at what his creation is doing. His huge head peers in through the dome, life-sized to my miniature. He's observing me like he would a creature in the undergrowth, with no less awe and wonder. I'm climbing upwards through soil, fossils, and layers of rock, past thousands of years of the bones of evolution. I've got to make it to the top, to the present, evolved and conscious, the winner of the human race.

On the surface of the earth the Chinese are invading. A huge army of giant monks marches westwards ethereally, like astronauts on the moon. They're dressed in white cotton crossover tunics and wide drawstring trousers, martial artists carrying weapons of mass construction: armed with formidable powers of the mind. Towering above me, they almost float they're so enlightened.

Mum and Dad visit. I'm full of regret for having dragged them down from their holiday in Scotland, again. It's Dad's favourite country and they usually head up the west coast, hiking and bird-watching. I drift off, still sensing them in the room. Hiding under the bed sheet, I make myself a cocoon. I'm just a foetus now and with every breath I expand into the womb I've made. I've got nine months to cook.

* * *

The communal area backs onto meadows and woodland, in the countryside not far from Bristol Airport. Patients seem to wander around aimlessly. There's a dark-skinned woman with tattoos and piercings. She looks Maori and is sitting on a bench just outside the back door. She seems familiar but I know we've never met before. Not in this life, anyway. I approach her slowly as she smokes outside the day room. Squatting down I reach up and gently take the gold stud from beneath her bottom lip into my mouth. It doesn't belong on her face. I think she calls for a nurse because one arrives pretty quickly and swiftly moves me away.

I head for the courtyard, a paved circular shaped area. A Somalian guy stands in the centre, his lower lip drooped and one hand skilfully flicking a cigarette lighter around. I walk quietly up to him and reach out to touch it. A soft layer of energy, blanketing him an inch or so above his skin, lets me in. I delicately stroke the gunmetal casing, which he stops playing with. Our feet take tiny steps anticlockwise, pivoting in a circle, like a dance. Facing each other, with our eyes looking down at our hands, we rotate slowly around the axis that is his lighter for a few moments before letting go.

A fenced-off area cuts across the far left hand corner of the garden. Loud music and voices beyond the flimsy wooden panels arouse my curiosity. I find a tiny slit between the slats and squint, trying to get a glimpse inside. There's a rectangular paved area in front of a red brick, single-storey building. Two people are sitting on the ground, with their backs against the wall. The man is bald and reminds me of Sol. The woman is younger, with bleached hair growing out at the roots. She reminds me of Zanna as she rolls a cigarette. An old transistor blares out

Radio One. They look like they're at a party and I want to go in. I walk along the fence searching for a door, but it's locked.

* * *

On the fourth day I'm moved into another room in a locked-off wing in the High Dependency Unit. Jenna slopes about in a wonky corset, the wrong buttonholes only half done-up. Her shoulders are slumped low and forwards and she looks me up and down with hatred as she walks past. She sucks back phlegm noisily and wipes her nose from hand to elbow for good measure. I feel like the new girl in the class, an unwelcome outsider. Jenna is the woman I saw hanging out with the bald guy behind the fence. The small concrete yard I first saw them both in is now my only access to the outdoors. They sit outside my bedroom window, shouting over the din of the radio. I've been allowed to join the party.

'Jesus is a rock in a sea of adversity,' a black guy calls out, like a Jamaican town crier chanting to the tune of *Come and Have a Go If You Think You're Hard Enough*. Two lines cut deeply into his cheeks, like grooves for tears.

Keith, the bald guy, heads over to the door in the fence and pushes some money through the gap by the lock. A small, folded square of white paper appears in its place and he takes it and puts it in his pocket. One of the nurses, with a wisp of fine grey bum fluff covering his otherwise bald head, looks like he wants to be in with the gang. Keith slips him the piece of paper from his pocket as they slide their palms together like brothers in the hood, covering up their illegal transaction. The man whose duty it is to make sure everyone takes their medication is, if I'm not mistaken, buying drugs from one of the patients.

My room contains the usual cupboard with no coat hangers, a bed and a sink. The overflow to the washbasin is filled with years of gunge. I want to clean it, but have nothing to use.

I lie back and fall into a deep reverie. Darkness and neon lights, businessmen, prostitutes, and bars in a red-light district. A Hong Kong drug ring moves cocaine and heroin via Bristol through festering pipes, clogged-up with the backlog of filth and grime and years of neglect, right into this hospital.

I open my eyes and turn onto my side, staring into the open wardrobe. I see a shape I can't quite make out. A faint purple and green light—a figure I don't recognise—is sitting in a chair inside, watching over me.

I close my eyes again and sense the presence of a woman behind peering over me, like a dentist.

'Are you sure you want to go through with this?' she asks.

'Absolutely.' I'm seeing whatever this is through to the end.

'Whatever the consequences?'

'Whatever the consequences.'

She ever-so-gently, without making an incision, removes the eggs from my ovaries one by one. I feel a small tug as each is pulled out. I guess that means I won't be having any children.

I peer down to the foot of my bed. My old English teacher, Mrs Richards, also purple and green light, is sitting in a chair looking at me. I don't notice if she's still wearing her usual beige Rohan walking trousers and plain white shirt. She doesn't speak out loud but I hear her thoughts. *Arrogant*, she thinks accusingly. Isn't that just like her to get me wrong?

Mrs Richards gave me three As in a row for my A Level English essays. The third one she initially graded A minus so I took it to her after class.

'I worked just as hard on this one as the other two and I'm wondering why you gave me an A minus for it.' I didn't really want to know. It was just my way of letting her know I'd rumbled her bullshit marking system. I was never an A student, and I was surprised I'd got As at all. I wasn't trying to get them. It was just how my essays turned out.

'Well I can't very well give you three As in a row now can I?' I gave her a hard stare that burned into her ridiculous logic. She took her pen and scrubbed out the minus. I didn't feel particularly arrogant, just fair. Am I being arrogant now, or is she just goading me?

* * *

Mum and Dad visit again. Dad tells me that there's been some discussion about my sectioning. I'm not aware I've been sectioned but that explains the move to the locked-off wing.

'When you arrived, you told the nurse you thought it was best if you were in hospital. She doesn't think you need sectioning. I've been fighting your case.'

There's usually no need to section someone who voluntarily admits themselves. My parents hate seeing me sectioned and don't think it's necessary. I'm not any danger to myself or anybody else. Dad tells me he had a meeting with the consultant psychiatrist to argue my case but they ended up in a confrontation.

'The fact that his medical opinion was being questioned', Dad says, 'ruffled his feathers. He insisted on keeping the sectioning in place just to pull rank because he claimed *he* was the expert.' He also made it clear that he had the power to administer me with electric shocks. It was said like a threat, to keep my dad in his place.

This hospital has a special locked ward for those who are sectioned. The other wards are open so patients can come and go as they please. The consultant as good as told Dad that it was costing a fortune paying for an agency nurse to be by my bed 24/7 on the main ward. It's cheaper to keep me under lock and key because it avoids extra staffing costs. It turns out my sectioning is purely a financial decision.

'I don't really care about being sectioned. But I need to touch the ground.'

'So you keep saying. One of the staff suggested we take you for a walk around the grounds. He thought it would do you good so they've agree to let you out with us.'

'Yeah, there's only a little concrete yard here. And there's only so many times I can trot around it.'

A wheelchair is brought for me. Now I'm not really sure if it's because I've said I can't use my legs today or whether the appearance of the chair makes me think I can't use them. I'm not really clear about the order of events but for some reason, I'm convinced I can't walk. Mum and Dad take it in turns to push me along the small lane that winds through the shaded woodland, past disused buildings in need of repair.

This place was built in the 1930s, to relieve the pressure on the overcrowded Victorian hospitals in the nearby city of Bristol. It was designed to create both a sense of privacy and community with clusters of villas built strategically to take advantage of the surrounding woodland. Before it was properly finished, it was commandeered by the Royal Navy at the outbreak of the Second World War. Maybe it has a lot of traumatised casualties of war still roaming around the corridors.

'Dad. How do you know I'm not dead?' Being dead might explain why I keep seeing spirits and disappearing into strange worlds.

'That's easy,' he says. 'I know you're not dead because dead people don't need to eat.' My dad is helpful like that: logical, calm, and strong. I think about his answer and it makes sense. I'll just have to find another explanation for the weirdness.

* * *

Having been free of episodes for six years, I've now experienced two in a row, only a year apart. And worse still, I've been sectioned. The Mental Health Act of 1983 is an Act of Parliament, which provides the legislation by which people diagnosed with a 'mental disorder' can be detained in hospital for assessment or treatment against their wishes. Incarceration, without trial, of people who have usually not committed any crime: those labelled as mentally ill are denied the rights afforded to all other citizens—with the possible exception of suspected terrorists.

Someone with a mental health problem is much more likely to be a victim than a perpetrator of violent crime. Even more worrying is that people with mental health problems are more of a danger to themselves than they are to others. Ninety per cent of people who die through suicide in the UK are experiencing mental distress.

In the state that I'm in right now, though, I couldn't care less about the implications of any of this. I head outside for my morning walk, round and round the courtyard, changing direction, making a figure of eight. I prance like my old friend Danielle and I used to do when we were growing up, impersonating a horse around a dressage arena.

It's a clear, sunny day so, when I'm done, I sit myself in a chair facing the rising sun. Derek Wilson—I see from his NHS name badge—comes over to join me and stands by my side. He waits a while before speaking.

'Whoops. There she goes. The bluebird of happiness, over the moon and under the stars.' He waves his hand through the air, arcing it away from me, his fingers fluttering. It's exactly what Michael Caine did in the movie *Little Voice*.

Michael Caine's character was quite the arsehole, pushing LV, or Little Voice, to sing in public when her singing was only ever a way to connect with her deceased dad. He exploits her talents and her traumatised state. Derek Wilson is copying the bit where Michael Caine tries to manipulate LV into wanting to perform so that Michael's character can benefit and get rich. I doubt quoting a dodgy character in a movie was ever on this guy's nurse-training syllabus. I give him an incredulous look. The staff on this wing are, in my opinion, worse than the patients.

Keith, the patient who reminds me of Solomon, comes outside into the yard, sits in a chair diagonally opposite me, and looks me right in the eyes. I look back questioningly. He grimaces and folds his arms across his chest, leaning back in his seat, inviting a challenge. I fold mine low across my belly protectively, bending forwards slightly.

He laughs like a pantomime villain. We remain staring into each other's eyes for a long time. My palms begin to itch and I rub them to relieve the irritation. Keith sees this as a victory and laughs again but I keep my gaze fixed firmly on him. As long as he's looking at me, I look back. I don't know what else to do. I scratch my reddening hands. How long is he going to keep this up? Eventually a member of staff walks by and Keith turns away to talk to him.

The next day a Bristol media friend of mine visits. She has gorgeous curly blonde hair and an open face. It must take some guts to come here, especially on your own. Though I originally know her from TV as a scriptwriter, she's also been doing a massage course and doesn't really feel comfortable in that world any more.

'I've brought you a gift.' She gives me a small brown paper bag with a Neal's Yard logo on. I open the blue glass bottle and smell the rose and geranium essential oil hand-cream before showing her my palms, which are now peeling.

'That's amazing,' I say. 'It's just what I needed.' Then I tell her about Keith and the primitive stand off we had, enjoying my impression of his bad boy act.

'His energy went right through me and made my hands itch like hell. My skin is actually peeling off now! Wow! You must have been really tuned in to me to have got me this.'

Of all the presents she could have brought, she's given me the only thing I really need.

* * *

I'm moved again, out of High Dependency Unit and back onto the main ward. I'm sharing a room with another woman around my age. She's got that gormless look of someone who's heavily medicated.

'Are you speaking in code?' she asks me from across the other side of room.

'No, I'm not,' I reply firmly, looking at her squarely so there's no doubt. I've pondered the same question myself but somehow I know not to ask people. It's unnerving being on the receiving end so I head downstairs to find a nurse.

'I'd like to move rooms. The woman I'm sharing with is freaking me out.' Without any fuss she sorts out another bed for me.

I gather my things and move back into the room I started in. I've come full circle.

CHAPTER TWELVE

Awakening

The central Bristol library, just off College Green, is always busy. Rows and rows of computers are available for two-hour slots. I come here to use the internet, as I don't have a computer at home. I'm normally researching and pitching documentary ideas to commissioning editors but today I'm searching for answers, as I get no help from the mental health services. Hospitalisation and medication is all they provide. I type 'spiritual' and 'psychosis' into the search engine and click on the first link. I don't know what I'm looking for exactly.

I'm taken to the home page of the Spiritual Emergency Network (SEN) in the States, which was founded in 1980 by Christina and Stanislav Grof in response to the lack of understanding and respect for psychospiritual growth in the mental health profession. So far, so good. I read the blurb which describes a sudden, intense, and overwhelming spiritual awakening that's too much for a person to cope with, when a spiritual emergence becomes an emergency.

It describes a spiritual emergency as a crisis often resulting in intense emotions, unusual thoughts and behaviours, and perceptual changes, which involves a spiritual component—such as experiences of death and rebirth, unity with the universe, and encounters with powerful beings. Among other things, it says that spiritual emergencies may be triggered by lack of sleep or deep spiritual practice or meditation. This fits me perfectly and I feel like they're describing exactly what I've been through.

'People experiencing these are often misdiagnosed with mental illness, like psychosis.'

As soon as I read this sentence, I burst into tears at the mistreatment I've received. I don't even care if people are looking at me I'm so engrossed. I order their book, *The Stormy Search for the Self*.

When the Grofs' book arrives, I open it immediately. By the third page I'm once again in floods of tears.

'One may suddenly experience the world as a manifestation of one cosmic, creative energy; nothing is separate. In the other, hidden realms are opened so that one encounters beings, deities, spirit guides and other wonderful or frightening forms or dimensions. These realms are not opinion but fact to those who have experienced them. Unfortunately, an individual with such an encounter will likely be labelled "psychotic" and prescribed tranquilizers by all but transpersonal practitioners. In mainstream medicine, there is no official recognition of the mystical truths or encounters underlying the religions of the world.'

Both psychotic and spiritual experiences involve escaping the limiting boundaries of the self, which leads to immense elation and freedom as the outlines of the confining selfhood melt down. But spiritual emergencies may actually be a natural developmental process rather than an illness, like psychosis. A spiritual emergency—if managed and treated under supervision—can, therefore, be life-changing and offer the individual a deeper sense of passion, wisdom, love, and zest for life, an expanded world view and overall improved feeling of well-being.

I devour the book, feeling a longing pulling inside me. I want my episodes to be welcomed by people. I want to be acknowledged for the depths to which I go to inside myself. If only there was a Spiritual Emergency Network in the UK.

* * *

Spark is Bristol's 'What's On' magazine for the alternative scene. It's free so I flick through it now and again. On this occasion an article jumps out at me because it's about spiritual emergencies. This coincidence happens only a few days after I've just found out about them. It's written by a woman based in Stroud, called Catherine Lucas. She wants to set up a

Spiritual Emergency Network in the UK and is interested to hear from readers. Talk about prayers being answered. I'm not the only one who gets in touch with her. Two others from Bristol also contact Catherine so she arranges to meet us all at the Boston Tea Party on Park Street.

The café is a trendy place, with stripped wooden floors, and tables and chairs that look like they've been commandeered from churches, country kitchens, and old school classrooms. It's busy, but we find a table in an upstairs corner. After exchanging personal stories Catherine tells us her plans.

'I'm organising a Revisioning Mental Health Conference at Hawkwood College in Stroud. The keynote speaker will be David Lukoff, who's coming from the States.' David, Catherine explains, is a transpersonal psychotherapist who's managed to get a new category added to the *DSM-IV*, the American *Diagnostic and Statistical Manual of Mental Disorders*. It means that 'religious or spiritual problem' can now be given as an official diagnosis. Does this mean I can now be diagnosed properly?

Finding the Spiritual Emergency Network in the US and the Spiritual Crisis Network in the UK is a game-changer. It validates all that I've been through: seeing auras, the orb of light, my healing hands, communicating with spiritual beings, visions of ancestors and other spirits are all reframed into a more positive light. Information from these organisations helps me dare to believe that my experiences are not a sign of insanity but some kind of shift in perception: a non-ordinary state of reality.

* * *

Hawkwood College is set in a nineteenth-century Grade II listed building, with idyllic gardens and sustainably managed land overlooking the Stroud Valley. Participants at this Revisioning Mental Health Conference range from academics, to mental health professionals, to personal experiencers, like me.

I make my way into the library for the welcoming tea. Most people are gathered around a central coffee table. An older gentleman has everyone's attention.

'I had one patient who would only respond to ECT. I never wanted to administer it but it's the only thing that ever worked on her. It brought her back to life for a while and then every so often we'd have to zap her again.' I recoil at his words. He must be a psychiatrist. I pick up one of his flyers. It turns out that Dr Adam Sinclair is the founder of something called the Society for the Release of Spirit Attachment. They believe that some mental disturbances are caused by spirits who are attached to people. They help to release the spirits, freeing the person from their symptoms. This is my kind of conference.

I regret skimping on the single accommodation supplement when my roommate snores, rumbling like an elephant's grief. I grab my pillow and duvet and head downstairs and curl up on the sofa in the lounge area. I'm a little wired from the excitement of the arrival and wound up by the snoring, but I manage to get a little sleep. In the morning, when I tell the staff where I spent the night, they give me my own room at no extra cost.

David Lukoff's talk is a very honest and personal account of his own spiritual emergency. He describes a personal crisis he went through after graduate school, when he decided to drop out and hitch around the States. One night, he saw a light shining from his hand, which had taken the shape of a mudrā, a symbolic, ritual hand gesture in the Buddhist and Hindu traditions. He thought it meant he was the reincarnation of the Buddha and Jesus, and felt he was to be the prophet of a new religion. He had conversations in his head with all kinds of people: Buddha and Christ, Locke and Rousseau, Freud and Jung, even Bob Dylan and Cat Stevens. He spent about five days, hardly sleeping, writing a holy book, which he photocopied and sent to his friends and family before handing it out to strangers on the street.

'I've no idea what happened to that book but I'm pretty sure it wasn't going to change the world,' he says, mocking himself slightly. Fortunately, he wasn't hospitalised and friends took care of him for a couple of months, until he returned to a more normal state.

'But I was left with a lot of questions. Why did a Jewish boy, who knew nothing about Buddhism or Christianity, have these feature so highly?'

So he read Carl Jung and Joseph Campbell, who described Christ as the archetype of the ideal self. He made sense of it all through therapy and went on to become a psychologist. At the end of his talk, he opens up the floor for questions. After some discussion, a woman with long wispy hair, parted down the middle, stands up.

'I lost my son.' She silences the room with her grave tone.

'I brought him up in a very liberal way, protecting him from the outside world as much as possible. We lived on the land, wild and free and he was very sensitive and creative.' She pauses to take a breath. 'He was going through a crisis and wasn't behaving in a way that society sees as acceptable, and he ended up getting arrested, and the police sectioned him. He was terrified, so he ran away. They chased after him but in trying to escape he hit his head on a steel girder and died.'

My throat closes up. Nobody speaks.

'If I hadn't sheltered him from the world so much then maybe he would have been more prepared to deal with it.'

She's brought into the room the gravity of the issue: people who are opening up to unusual dimensions that are scary and unfamiliar need a different kind of help to what the mental health services provide. Lives are at stake.

Someone else introduces Jung's idea of the shadow. They get quite passionate drawing a diagram on a whiteboard to show that a spiritual emergency is all of the stuff we've hidden away down in the murky depths of our psyche coming up to be dealt with. The more you have hidden away: negative emotions, negative impulses, traumatic memories, etc., the more undigested psychological material there is to deal with. So if it is a form of spiritual awakening, it's not just about love and light. It's more like a light being shone on the darkness.

Discovering that I was sexually abused is a perfect example of accessing this unconscious, or shadow. I had no idea I'd been abused until I made some claims during my first episode. The part of me that knew it to be true, that is, my unconscious, had become conscious.

Carl Jung established a school of psychology that emphasises a quest for wholeness. This he saw as the integration of the conscious with the unconscious. He also talked about archetypal figures as highly developed elements of the collective unconscious. Jung included religious figures among these archetypes. The devil, he claimed, is a character within each of us, as is Jesus, who represents our idealised self. Accessing these archetypes within is seen as a necessary process which is essential in order to return to wholeness. Having had both Jesus and devil figures appear to me during my so-called psychosis, I wonder if I'm just tapping into this collective unconscious.

Later that evening, the grieving mother joins us for the 5Rhythms dance event. While everyone else is moving their bodies to the music, the woman with the long wispy hair parted down the middle races around, winding in and out of people, her arms above her head, wailing loudly. If you didn't know she was mad with grief, you would think she was just plain mad.

The next day I sign up for a Family Constellation workshop. I don't know what this is but I'm curious about the idea behind it. Apparently, when there's a secret in the family tree, like a mysterious death that was never acknowledged, the ancestral spirit can cause disturbances in the people alive today in order to be known. The soul cannot rest when it has experienced an unjust or violent death. They try to get through via the most open and sensitive family member, which can show up as psychosis. It requires a belief in the existence of our spirit or soul surviving after death so this is not a mainstream concept. But then again, this conference is no mainstream kind of conference.

One person is going to be selected to explore their lineage. They will have to choose other participants to represent each member of their family, alive and dead, as far back as they can. The lucky person has to place their relatives intuitively in the space. Jewish people, for example, often place them all spread far and wide randomly, reflecting the displacement that has occurred in their ancestral line.

To begin with, we sit in a large circle and the woman facilitating leads us in a guided meditation.

'Imagine your ancestors all standing behind you, ever increasing rows of grandparents and great-grandparents. All the way back.'

I didn't really know my grandparents. Most of them died before I was born. The only one I did know, I hardly ever saw because we were living overseas. My grandfather, on my dad's side, was a musician and travelled the world playing the organ on cruise ships. When he lived with us for a while, when I was about eight years old, he taught me the cha-cha. He was a quiet man and sat in the same chair all day reading the newspaper.

I can't picture them all behind me. I don't really know what any of the others look like. Instead I jump up above the surface of the earth and fly across the planet seeing how all the people of the world are interconnected, if you go back far enough.

When we're finished, we each have to share our experience with the group. I'm embarrassed to tell everyone about mine because it's so different from the others.

'Emma ...' The facilitator turns to me once everyone has spoken. 'You describe exactly the kind of energy I'd like to work with today. Would you like to step in and work with me?'

I'm taken aback but I get up and stand in the middle of the circle and wait for her instructions.

'Look around the room and pick out people to represent your family.'

I examine everyone in turn. There's a woman that looks kind of motherly but she looks nothing like my mum. A short, dark-haired male could be my father but again he doesn't look anything like him. I'm a little frozen. I think my head is getting in the way of picking anybody out.

'I can't do it,' I tell her, hoping she'll give me the encouragement I need.

'OK. I trust that your soul isn't ready for whatever reason and it's not the right time. Sit down and we'll let someone else have a go.'

I'm relieved, but also disappointed, and annoyed with myself. This woman has come from Germany and she's clearly leading the way with this work. But perhaps I'm not ready for what it might uncover.

After the conference, I join the board of trustees of the Spiritual Crisis Network. I also volunteer on their email rota, which acts like a helpline. I discover lots of other people who are going through a similar thing. They contact the SCN for support. Some people are avoiding treatment from the mental health services, while others are trying to find a way to break free from them. We can't do much except validate their experiences and suggest ways they could ground themselves.

As long as I'm around people who are convinced their non-ordinary state of reality is real, I feel more certain of my own. But my parents don't buy the whole spiritual interpretation and never will. Despite that, they still make a regular donation to the Spiritual Crisis Network as a show of support. It's difficult to maintain my conviction when I'm around people who believe there is no spiritual dimension.

I turn to the internet again for some reassurance. My online search reveals an article citing a large number of monks in China that went mad from doing too much *qigong*. The rationale was that gathering large amounts of *chi* into the body caused the old stagnant energy to be released into the system. This is like adding too much fresh water into a stagnant, old reservoir, breaking the dam, releasing the festering swamp and contaminating the rest of the water supply. It's kind of similar to shining the light on the darkness. New *chi* pushing out the old. According to this website I'm a '*qigong* casualty'.

EPISODE FOUR

CHAPTER THIRTEEN

Soulmate

R ows and rows of self-help books surround me on three sides. On the fourth, a large display unit corrals me into the corner of Waterstones bookshop, blocking me in but conveniently hiding me from the other shoppers. This is not a section I want to be seen in. I'm drawn to one paperback in particular, *Finding Your Soul Mate*. The name 'Michael' is printed across the cover. Was the author too embarrassed to put his full name to it? I read the back cover, despite my cynicism, while the gremlin on my left shoulder mocks me.

You can't buy this! It's a load of rubbish.

I put the book back in its place and slide my forefinger gently over the spines of others, searching for something more acceptable. I pull out another on the same subject and the gremlin on my right rolls its eyes.

If you're going to get that one you may as well get the other! It's the one you really want.

A little embarrassed, I hand my card over at the till and hope the assistant, a young man, doesn't notice what it's about, before heading straight home to indulge myself. It's an easy read and by the end of the afternoon, I've already finished it. I flick back through the pages to find the chapter on how to put it into practice.

First I make a list of all the qualities I want my soulmate to possess. Then I have to give a date by which I'd like to meet him. I settle for the end of the year. It's April 2005 and it feels realistic. An excited little gremlin is jumping up and down.

A week! Within a week, please!

Over the initial resistance, I wholeheartedly throw myself into the process. Every day, at the same time, I look out of my bedroom window and send out a message to *him*.

I'm here! My name is Emma. I live in Princes Place, Bishopston, Bristol. I'm waiting for you. Please come and find me. We'll go for lovely walks together in wild places and cook gorgeous food and see amazing films. I'm ready for you.

Exactly a week later, I glide down the street in my bright red wool coat to do my shopping, knowing with every fibre of my being that I'm going to meet my soulmate very soon. I don't have to do anything different or go anywhere in particular to find him. It's a relief I can just get on with my life as normal.

Gloucester Road is one of the most diverse high streets in the country. I stopped going to supermarkets earlier this year because I made a new year's resolution to use less plastic. Nearly everything in the supermarket is packaged in it. It revolutionised how I shop. Now I go to my local independent greengrocer, butcher, and baker, who are all, luckily, right on my doorstep.

I start at the far end, in Harvest Health Food shop, to refill my washing-up liquid. I retrieve the empty plastic container from my bag-for-life, unscrew the top, and squat down in front of the large refill barrel. I sense a guy hovering behind me. *Is he checking me out?* I push down the tap, holding my used bottle with some concentration.

'You have a very steady hand,' the man compliments me.

'Last time I spilt it everywhere, so I'm being extra careful.'

When it's full, he's still hanging around, not really attending to his shopping. He's very tall, wears glasses, about my age, and has a full head of mousy brown hair, like mine. He's not bad-looking, if a little intellectual and geeky, like a dashing head-boy type.

'Excuse me.' I shimmy past him to get to the grain coffee on the shelf he's pretending to look at before going to the counter to pay. I can tell he can't concentrate on his shopping, even though he's trying to look like he's not paying me any attention.

Next up, the bakery, a few doors down, where there's a queue. There's always a queue because they make proper bread that is worth waiting for. I get my sourdough loaf and turn to go. The guy from the health food shop is now waiting at the back of the line.

'Hello again,' I smile knowingly.

'Hello,' he says back and then I continue down the street.

Out of the corner of my eye I see a long pair of legs stretching to get to a parked car I'm about to walk past. There's no way he's been served and finished in the bakery in that short amount of time. No, he's rushing so as not to miss me. He makes it just as I'm about to walk past and leans against the driver's door in a forced laid-back pose.

'Hello,' he says smiling. 'Have we met before?' I want to say *duh, yeah, in the health food shop, and then you were stalking me in the bread shop* but I go along with his obvious pretence, opting for a less teasing option to save his face.

'I live around here, so maybe you've seen me about.'

'Yeah. Maybe.' He looks dissatisfied but drops the subject. 'I'm Ciaran,' he says holding his hand out for a formal introduction.

'I'm Emma,' I say, shaking it. 'Hopefully see you around.' I genuinely mean it and continue on my way to the greengrocer, 100 yards or so further up. Just as I'm approaching, the same car pulls in a few metres ahead of me. Ciaran gets out and turns to face me.

'Hello,' he greets me.

'Hello again,' I reply with joke suspicion.

'Do you want to go out for coffee sometime?' he asks bravely.

'OK,' I reply, throwing caution to the wind, and we exchange mobile numbers.

Later that same afternoon, as I'm heading back from my swim, a guy walking on the opposite side of the road looks across at me and I smile back.

'Hey,' he says, flicking his head slightly.

'Hi,' I say in return. He crosses over with a limping gait that some guys must think looks cool.

'Where you headed?' he asks, walking alongside me.

'Home. I live just off Gloucester Road,' I say, nudging my head towards the junction. 'What about you?'

'Off to college. Doin' a photography course.'

'I've been doing some photography,' I respond, to make a connection.

'Wow. Cool,' he says, a little over the top, as if the coincidence is really amazing. 'What you been photographin'?'

'Tree bark.'

We reach the junction where he says he's turning right and he stops and asks me for my number. Twice in one day. No one has ever stopped me on the street and asked me for my number before. The book is definitely working, but I wasn't expecting to have to choose between two soulmates.

I have a small back garden, quite large for a terraced house and I spend a lot of time tending it. It's a love/hate relationship: I love what it could be, but hate that it's never finished. My phone rings and I wipe the dirt off my hands to answer it.

'Hi. It's Ciaran,' he says, gently.

'Hi Ciaran. How are you?' I put the trowel down and lean against the shed door.

'I've just been to the dentist and the left side of my face is a bit numb so sorry if I sound funny.'

'I hate going to the dentist,' I say in sympathy. 'I only go once every five years for a check-up.'

'How are you? What are you up to?' he asks.

'I'm good, thanks. I'm just doing some gardening.'

'I run a gardening project on the Redcliffe estate.'

'Is that what you do for a living?' I hadn't pegged him as a gardener. He's not the rugged-looking type.

'Only part-time. It helps pay the bills. I'm a writer.'

'Wow, you're a writer? What do you write?'

'Well, I've got a Radio Four play coming up.'

'I'm impressed. That's hard to break into.'

'Yeah. It was.' Ciaran pauses. 'Anyway, I'm calling to arrange our coffee.'

'Great,' I say. 'Where do you suggest?'

'Do you know La Ruca?'

'Is that the café above the shop on Gloucester Road? I've not been but I've always wondered about it.'

'Yes. Are you free for breakfast on Saturday morning? I'm really busy this week and that's my only window.'

'What time?'

'9 o'clock?'

'OK. See you then.'

This guy obviously doesn't go mashing it up on a Friday night. I like that he's fitting me in even though he's clearly got a full schedule.

The next day my phone pings with a text coming in.

How R U Do In? When Can We Hook Up?

It's the other guy. I don't like his way of communicating, or putting the onus onto me of when we meet. Texts like this are going to bug the shit out of me and I don't think I want to juggle two men at once. I tell him I've changed my mind and he doesn't sound too happy about it.

We Cudda Had Amazin Adventures 2gether.

I think I've made the right choice.

The first date with Ciaran gives me an opportunity to check him out a little. He's quite intense and serious-looking. The glasses don't help. I'm not immediately drawn to him, but I'm not getting a big 'no' either.

'You're studying shiatsu? I'm a shiatsu practitioner!' he says, happily surprised.

'Really? Wow! How long have you been practising?'

'About ten years. I went to the Shiatsu College, London and work at the Relaxation Centre now.'

'Really?' I say again. 'Do you know Annabel? She's on my shiatsu course and does massage there.'

'Yeah. I know Annabel. Small world.' Ciaran smiles.

He walks me home through the back streets and I tell him how I'm looking for my soulmate. I'm thirty-five and am done messing around. I want the whole deal and I'm not playing games or following those stupid dating rules that tell you not to scare men off by mentioning marriage on the first date. I figure if the idea of a soulmate freaks him out then I'm not interested in him anyway.

His tallness is strange to walk beside. His six foot four to my five foot four means I'm talking to his chest. We turn into my cul-de-sac and stop at my little wrought iron gate. I'm not sure if he's hoping I'll invite him in. For me the date is over and I'm guessing there'll be another one. Ciaran pushes for some kind of confirmation of my interest. It feels way too soon to know how I feel about him. I'm not *not* interested. I wasn't expecting the third degree on my feelings on our first date and feel backed into a corner. When I don't give him the reassurance he's looking for he pushes harder. I'm not going to be allowed to say goodbye without giving him some clarity so I decide to be honest. A bit too honest.

'I'm not physically attracted to you,' I say, with my northern bluntness.

'That was difficult to hear.' He looks hurt so I offer him some encouragement.

'I like the way you just said that it was difficult to hear. You obviously have great communication skills.'

We say goodbye and Ciaran texts me the next day.

'What's attraction like for you? Is it an immediate thing, or does it grow?'

'I've no idea. Maybe it will grow, maybe it won't.'

The second date feels easier and takes place in the evening, giving us more time. Ciaran's place is only fifteen minutes walk from mine. It's a big house on Sydenham Road and he greets me at the door with a cute smile. I'm impressed. Houses in this area are not cheap.

'It's not my house. I rent the flat on the top floor. Martha and Max are lovely but their kids are all grown-up and they don't need all this space.'

We make our way up the three flights of stairs, through Martha and Max's to the top floor. Ciaran's been cooking and various utensils are discarded in the sink.

'I'm making a salmon dish. Do you eat fish?'

'I love it! Do you enjoy cooking?'

'Yeah. I could have been a chef, but I didn't want to spoil my love of food. It's very stressful in catering, the time-pressure and stuff.'

The meal is well presented, Ciaran taking care to lay it all out beautifully.

'Wow. I just throw it all on the plate.'

'If I've made a nice meal, I like to serve it with care and attention.'

I wash up after we've finished, as a show of appreciation and Ciaran puts on some music. I recognise the acid jazzy intro of St Germain, *I want you to get together*. The words set off a nervous reaction in my body. I'm pretty sure Ciaran's not aware of the message in the song because most men don't really listen to lyrics. Having his unconscious serenading me makes me feel quite uneasy. To make matters worse, it's the only words in the song and they just keep repeating. I clam up and focus on washing the pots, hoping my anxiety will pass.

When I turn around, Ciaran is watching me. He reaches out and takes my hand, holding a pressure point. He's plugged into Large Intestine 4, just in the webbing between my thumb and forefinger. It's a letting-go point and I feel my energy thumping back down into my body with a clunk.

'What's happening?' he asks, still holding the point.

'I'm scared.' I pause before asking him why he went for that point.
'Intuition, I suppose. I didn't really think about it.' My fear subsides,
leaving me with admiration. Ciaran seems to know just what I need and
I like that. Here's a man who could be good for me. His skill as a shiatsu
practitioner will be useful. I look more closely at his features. He's not
wearing glasses today and his hazel eyes are clear and attractive. In fact
his whole face is rather easy on the eyes. I hadn't really noticed before
because I couldn't see him for his glasses.

* * *

We've been dating for a month now and it's going quite well. Ciaran's
a gifted writer and very driven. He and his friend used to put on liter-
ary events so they could perform their work in public. It was just a
ruse so he could get his talent spotted. They invited all sorts of people
to attend, including a Radio Four producer who was impressed with
Ciaran's stories and commissioned him to write a play. I know how
hard it is to break into the broadcasting world. It takes self-belief, perse-
verance, and an ability to sell yourself. It's hard to imagine he once had
a drug problem.

Ciaran grew up in west London with his dad, his parents having
split up when he was a baby. His mother was the main caregiver, to
begin with, but when her new boyfriend made her choose between him
and her son, she left Ciaran with his dad. Ciaran's dad was an actor
and hung out with a few famous people but mostly earned his living
through drug-dealing. He was also involved in bank robbery, as the get-
away driver. This meant he was in and out of prison leaving Ciaran with
a stepmother who, fortunately, loved him unconditionally and treated
him like her own. But it also left him vulnerable; to being groomed by
the caretaker of the apartment they lived in, who sexually abused him
when he was only twelve years old. He went downhill after that and
ended up on heroin by the time he was sixteen. When he was arrested,
the judge offered him a choice: prison or rehab. So on his twenty-first
birthday, Ciaran went into rehab and he's been clean ever since.

Ciaran can't wait to show me around the council estate garden he
manages and proudly points out all the bits he's helped to create. It's
a concreted area around high-rise flats with the occasional raised bed
looking very out of place. They have to collect a lot of litter and used
needles that lie around the dark corners. This community project looks

like a do-gooder's sticking plaster on a burst artery of a social problem and I can't wait to get away. The people walking around are hunched over and scowl at me unwelcomingly.

We head to the nearby St Mary Redcliffe Church and Ciaran lays out a blanket on the grass for us to sit on. He's brought lots of goodies for a picnic lunch. While I'm tucking into hummus, crackers, and olives, Ciaran hands me a letter, which I think a little strange considering he's sitting right in front of me.

'Shall I read it now?'

'If you like.'

I open it and read it silently to myself. It says that he wants to have a relationship with me but feels he needs to be honest so we can embark on one without lies. It goes on to say that while I was away at the weekend he slept with some woman or other who'd been interested in him but he wasn't really interested in her. He knew it was a mistake and felt it wasn't an infidelity because we weren't yet in a relationship. The rest of the letter is a wordy attempt to try to control my reaction. I feel kicked in the stomach.

'I know we haven't yet defined our relationship but it *feels* like an infidelity to me.' I look deep into his eyes to see what I can find there. He's afraid. We've been meeting up a couple of times a week, mostly in neutral territory, getting to know each other. We haven't rushed into sex and have only kissed briefly while we were out for a walk. I felt that we were getting closer, and was happy for things to progress naturally. The realisation that he sleeps with women he's not actually interested in comes as a shock. I guess this is the impact that his traumatic childhood has had on him.

I tell him I need some time to think, as I can't make a decision right now. It seems like a strange way to broach the subject of getting into a relationship but I keep that to myself.

'Take all the time you need,' Ciaran says. I walk home alone, feeling confused and disappointed.

I decide to talk to a few friends to get their opinion in the hope that it will help me come to a decision. Annabel, the shiatsu friend who knows Ciaran from her massage work at the Relaxation Centre, is very much against a relationship with him.

'If he's like that now then it's a bad sign, and it really doesn't bode well for the future does it?'

Eleanor is a little more sympathetic. She's another fellow shiatsu student who also happens to know Ciaran, through a support group they both go to. She refuses to make any judgements about him and that makes me feel less black-and-white about it. It makes me think about his upbringing, and how it might have affected him.

Is he a liability, or does he—like everyone—deserve a second chance? I weigh up the situation from every angle but ultimately I think Annabel is right, it doesn't bode well for the future. After two days of inner turmoil and deep soul-searching, I make up my mind. I call round to Ciaran's flat to give him an answer. I walk up the three flights of stairs silently, feeling calm, grounded, and clear about my decision. We head into the kitchen-slash-living room, and I don't bother with small talk.

'I've thought a lot about this situation, Ciaran, and consulted friends for their opinion as well.' I pause and look him directly in the eyes. 'I've decided not to get into a relationship with you.'

Ciaran turns away and walks into his bedroom. I don't know what he's gone to scrabble around in there for. I think he's hurt and needs to get away. I hear a smash of something accidentally broken.

'That was the vase of tulips you gave me,' he says with a tone that tells me it's my fault.

I laugh. Partly to relieve the tension and partly because it's so ironic. I gave him the tulips as a romantic gesture. I'd been to a wedding in Cornwall and afterwards we were all encouraged to take home the flowers from the tables. That same weekend was when Ciaran slept with someone else. I don't believe in accidents. I think his unconscious mind makes him knock the vase over, breaking the container that was holding a representation of my love. Perhaps he needs this poetic drama to see it visually in order to feel it emotionally.

'It's not funny,' Ciaran yells through the walls. 'You're twisted if you think it's funny.'

'I'm going to go now, Ciaran.' I don't like how he's taking his pain out on me. He's behaving like a little child. I'm not staying to be his emotional punchbag but I have to go through his bedroom in order to get out of his flat. Ciaran is standing in the middle of it frozen, like a rabbit caught in the headlights.

'Goodbye, Ciaran,' I say softly. But he doesn't speak or maybe he can't. I walk slowly back downstairs and out of the front door, down the short path and through the little gate. I turn right, towards home, and head up the hill.

I'm not going to look back.

'*Ehhhh-mmaa!*' I hear my name shouted. I turn around, and Ciaran is standing at the gate. I go back down the hill and he squats down on the step so that he's almost level with me.

'Is there *anything* I can do?' He sounds pleading and genuine, like there's nothing he wouldn't do for me. I'm aware of how quickly he's turned himself around.

You just did it, I think to myself, before walking back into the house where we make our way back up the stairs to his little attic flat, together.

CHAPTER FOURTEEN

Priestess

It's Friday night and Annabel and I are having one of our irregular catch-ups that have become more regular since I've been seeing Ciaran. Annabel has beautiful long, curly brown hair and large doe eyes to match. She's one of those people who I could have easily known at school, with a youthfulness that doesn't age. Her head is in the clouds most of the time, in touch with the spiritual realm, so I like hanging out with her. She's different from my TV friends and I can talk freely about weird and wonderful spiritual stuff. She's telling me about this man she met recently called James Abraham. I raise my eyebrows questioningly—always thinking about men!

'No, it's not like that. He's old. He works with crystals.'

'I'm not really into crystals. I've never felt anything from them.'

'It's hard to describe what he does exactly. To say that he works with crystals just doesn't do it justice. He's like a shaman or something. After I met him I had this vision of us in Australia and it was really strong so I told him about it. He's totally in service and goes wherever spirit guides him. We're going to go and work with the energy lines around Uluru. He's really into healing the earth's energy.'

I'm intrigued and I want to meet him but dashing off to Australia sounds impulsive. I also don't think it's the earth that needs healing but mankind upon it!

'Anyway, how's it going with Ciaran?'

'Well, it was a rocky start, as you know. He's quite intense and I just kept letting go of it. But each time I do, something shifts and he just sort of snaps out of it. Like it breaks the mad spell he's under. I'm not sure whether I should just totally end it though. I'm feeling quite confused.'

'As you're speaking, I can see something weird coming out of your head.'

'Right,' I say, not sure if it's just her vivid imagination.

'I'm just gonna check with James if you don't mind.' She reaches for her mobile. 'Hi James. I'm sitting with my friend Emma and I can see these strange alien beings coming out of her head.' She pauses, listening to his response, then turns to me. 'James says can you come over now? It's pretty urgent.'

'Errr ... OK.' James is friendly but slightly panicked. He's not as old as I imagined or maybe it's his short, slim build that makes him seem younger. He has a friendly open face, despite looking a bit stressed and seems trustworthy enough. He shows me into a room with no furniture and asks me to lie on the floor. James and Annabel scurry around my feet whispering to each other. It doesn't feel right. Annabel's a bit naive and this guy's probably going to charge me a fortune.

'I'm feeling a bit freaked out,' I confess. 'I'm a bit paranoid that Annabel is like a gofer, a pawn you send out to get people and bring them to you.' They look at each other knowingly and then James turns to me.

'You're picking up something from a past life we all had together. I did some terrible things. I can't tell you about it now. It's too awful.'

Annabel holds my ankles and James frantically spins a chain with a crystal on the end.

'There are entities attached to you and they've harvesting your fear as an energy source.' He spins the pendulum again, as if waiting for the next bit of information. He looks quite distraught. 'There are thousands of people like you that they're feeding off.' I imagine he's talking about all the other people I've met on psychiatric wards. 'I work with the Archangel Michael. Do I have your permission to clear this?'

'Yes,' I reply, amused but curious.

James arranges his crystals on the floor around me according to the instructions he's receiving from his pendulum. One by one, he turns them 180 degrees clockwise. Annabel stays at the other end of the room, holding my feet.

'I'm just opening a gateway.' Then he chants something in what sounds like a totally made-up language.

'I feel like I've got chains around my ankles.'

'Don't worry,' James assures me. 'Annabel's just clearing another past life in which you were shackled.'

He carefully places a huge crystal bowl on my belly. With great ceremony and concentration, he taps the bowl with the striker and circles it around the rim. Its heavenly sound vibrates through my entire body as it sings out a long, pure note. A wave of tingles flood me, through my head, and down my arms and legs. It feels like I'm being cleaned from the inside.

'I ask the Lord Karma to clear away any past karma and cancel any future karma for all eternity.' I'm jolted out of my bliss. If karma exists, I'm pretty sure it's just cause and effect and cannot be cancelled. Who does this guy think he is? And is there even such a thing as Lord Karma?

'I've been working with the Ashtar Command, a group of beings that includes the Christ Consciousness. I've never worked with them before. They're assigned to you and you can ask for their help at any time. You just have to say Ashtar Command three times.' He pauses but I don't know what to say because I only half believe him. Part of me wants it to be true but the other half thinks it might be a load of bollocks.

'You are a High Priestess of Avalon,' James continues reverently. 'You should drink the waters of Glastonbury.' He puts the crystals away but keeps hold of the pendulum, offering me the opportunity to ask it a question. All I want to know about is my relationship with Ciaran.

'Is it in my highest interests to end my relationship with Ciaran?'

'Do I have permission from Ciaran on all levels to ask?' The pendulum swings rapidly around clockwise indicating the affirmative so he poses my question. It turns quickly again in the same direction.

'Yes,' he says looking up from his pendulum.

As I'm getting ready to go, I wonder how much he's going to charge me but I don't want to broach the subject.

'I normally charge for this work but for you I'm making an exception. Consider it a gift. I owe you.'

I'm not sure how much of it I believe, but I do feel taller and more expansive and I liked being told I was the High Priestess of Avalon. The thought of breaking up with Ciaran makes me feel guilty though.

What would I tell him? Some guy's pendulum told me to break up with you?

* * *

I pull into the Abbey car park and get a ticket from the machine. I've never been to Glastonbury before. It's full of crystal shops and rainbow jumpers, but it doesn't look right somehow alongside the Sixties' council blocks. I mooch around browsing shop windows and wondering if I could ever live here. I'd quite like to get out of the city.

I'm drawn to a noticeboard under an archway that leads into a cobbled courtyard. *Priestess of Avalon Training—Glastonbury Goddess Temple.* I'm taken aback. *I'm* the Priestess of Avalon. I laugh at my ego. I'm curious about the course but can't quite get past my feelings of superiority to write down the details.

I head to Wellhouse Lane to get what I came for. There are two spouts on either side of the road, small copper pipes in the walls that continuously flow with water from beneath Glastonbury Tor. On the left hand side is the red water, on the right, the white. There's somebody filling up from the white one so I put my bottle under the gushing spout on the left. When it's full, I take a sip. It tastes like blood. It must be the iron. I cross to the other side of the road where a drunk is sitting on a bench rolling a cigarette. He looks lined with age, poor living, and a painful past. I taste the white water. It's sweet and full of minerals.

Glastonbury is known for its festival but that actually takes place in a small village called Pilton a mile or two away. The town itself has attracted lots of hippies who appear to have come for the festival and never left. The place contains a lot of what I call pseudo-spirituality: people wearing nymph, goddess, and pixie-like clothes and spouting pseudoscience to back up all kinds of strange beliefs. It has its fair share of chronically sick people suffering with ME or drug addiction or mental health problems. I guess the healing waters and powerful history of the place make many people want to move here. There are legends of King Arthur being buried here and Joseph of Arimathea setting up the first church. I'm not sure I could live here though. I'm just not into all the tie-dyed robes and dreadlocks. The attitude is all 'one love' on the surface but a lot of that seems drug-fuelled to me.

* * *

Ciaran's moving in and it's freaking us both out. Neither of us has co-habited before but we've been together a year now so it seems like the next step. The week leading up to it, I bump into Sol in the shop down the road, which never happens. The actual interaction itself is nothing special but it feels epic, like the past clearing itself out to make way for the new.

I want to make space in my house for Ciaran, as a gesture of welcome, so he feels like it's his place too. I have a matching pair of large metal picture frames that have been filled with photos of me and my family and friends. I empty one of them and rearrange the other, placing a lovely shot of us both together right in the centre of it. I give the other one to Ciaran to fill with his own pictures.

Ciaran's been having a massive clear-out so as not to bring a load of junk with him. I find an old photograph that has fallen down between the arm and the seat of the sofa. Adrenalin shoots into my chest. A naked woman, kneeling with her legs closed, looks up at me. She has long curly hair and ample breasts. I rush outside to rifle through the paper recycling box thinking there's bound to be some more evidence of Ciaran's past in there. In a blind panic, I flick through some more photos that he's discarded as he was chucking his old stuff out. An image of a big, hard, veiny penis jumps out at me.

This is it! I've found it!

I pull it out for a better look, wondering at the same time why the hell I would want to see it more closely. My fear is playing tricks with me because it's not a penis at all but a man's neck. I pull myself together and resolve to ask Ciaran about the photo of the nude woman when he gets back from work.

I know he has a past that I'd rather not know the details of. I know he's already slept with someone else while we were first dating. I know he's likely to do it again, when he's struggling and forgets that the fix never fixes things. I know all this but I also believe in the power of people to change and he works really hard at it.

I look at the naked woman again. There's anger in her jutting-out jaw, and in her eyes there's a sadness that looks far away. She turns out to be an ex-girlfriend, unaware and unable to recognise the damage they are both doing to each other.

CHAPTER FIFTEEN

Initiation

T he following May, in 2006, my shiatsu course is coming to an end and it's marked by a residential, which takes place in an old mansion in a small village called Horrabridge, on Dartmoor. It's part and parcel of the three-year course and is an intense initiation process. I'm not sure what that means, but Ken is always keen to facilitate people to unblock negative thought patterns and emotions that hold us back from being the magnificent selves he thinks we were all born to be.

He's been doing this kind of work for over twenty years and loves it. He was part of the men's movement in the Eighties: Robert Bly and the East West Centre in London. He mostly focuses on freeing stuck emotions that we bury as a result of socialisation. I've noticed I've certainly got a lot of anger locked away and, beneath that, hurt and grief. He believes they are the root cause of many diseases as the energy block prevents the smooth flow of *chi*.

The evening of our arrival is spent settling in and setting the ground rules:

No side talking
Everything we say must be to the whole group
No leaving the room with our emotions

Emotions are to be expressed in front of everyone because going elsewhere is a form of attention seeking and drama

This is going to be an interesting week!

'We're staying in a separate wing of the house,' Ken explains, referring to himself, his partner Becky, and Matt McKenzie, the co-principal
of the school. 'And when we're over there, it's our private time and
we're not to be disturbed. Is that clear for everyone?'

'Can you make an exception for me? What if I have an episode? I
might have to come and disturb you.' Ken pauses before responding.

'OK, Emma. We'll make an exception.' Ken's response triggers one
of the other students.

'That's not fair. With the work that we're doing here, we're all vulnerable. Any one of us may get into difficulty and need to see you.' The
atmosphere is sullen and we're all a bit scared, to say the least, looking
for assurances. It's agreed that in emergencies anyone can enter their
section of the building.

Next we have an opening ceremony to set the intention for the week.
Ken reads a poem to kick it off. Healing, by D. H. Lawrence. It's not
a poem I'm familiar with and it's about how we get ill, not because
our various parts are not working properly, but because of emotional
wounds to the soul. In order to heal, we have to free ourselves from the
repetition of life's mistakes. My throat closes up on hearing the last line.
I don't know what mistakes I've been repeating but I intuitively understand that society applauds them.

We form a large circle, and invite whatever ancestors and spirits we
want to help us on this initiatory journey we're embarking on. One by
one, each student steps forward and calls out a name, then steps back,
rejoining the others.

'I'd like to call in the Ashtar Command. But I have to say it three times.'

'OK,' Ken says. 'Go ahead.'

I googled the Ashtar Command and discovered they're apparently a
group of beings, led by Commander Ashtar, who was known on earth
as Jesus. This information is supposedly channelled and they allegedly
claim to be helping humans with an ascension process, that is, a shift
from the physical dimension to the etheric. I'm not convinced of all of
this but I'd like it to be true.

'Ashtar Command. Ashtar Command. Ashtar Command,' I say,
feeling like an idiot but just in case they do exist, I want their help.

As I don't have any strong ties to my grandparents I can't think of any ancestors I'd like to have with me. They're all very down to earth people from Yorkshire and I imagine they would find this whole thing a bit weird anyway.

Then Becky takes charge and leads us all in a shaking exercise.

'Relax your wrists and shake out your hands. Really shake them. Now let your whole arm shake. Great. Do the same with your feet. And now your legs. Shake it all out. Shake your hips. Now let go of your whole body and shake. Shake everything out.' The room is a chaos of limbs and hair and blurredness. 'Shake out your stuckness. Shake out your resentment. Shake out your embarrassment.' My body tingles with energy dislodging from stagnant corners, which I flick out through my skin.

'Now I'm going to count backwards from ten. Trust that when I get to one, whatever needs to happen will happen.' Ken's taken over from Becky and the mood in the room shifts to one of fearful anticipation.

'What's going to happen?' a student asks, trying to grasp control.

'It'll be different for everyone. Trust that your soul knows.'

'What if I don't know what to do?'

'So much resistance,' I overhear Matt McKenzie whisper judgementally to one of the assistants so I jump to our defence.

'Yes, we all have our resistance, Matt. There's nothing wrong with that,' I say, making sure everyone else can hear me.

'If we're not supposed to side talk then I think that rule should apply to you too, Matt,' another brave student asserts. We're a feisty lot and I don't envy their role having to supervise.

'Just allow whatever comes through you to come through,' Ken continues, settling our nerves and refocusing our attention.

I stand still enjoying the feeling of the tingles dissipating as Ken counts down.

'Ten, nine, eight, seven, six, five, four, three, two, one.'

Someone must have pressed play on the stereo because the Tears for Fears song 'Shout' has come on full volume. People are screaming and shouting. I think they're manipulated by the music. I don't feel like shouting just because the lyrics say so. I don't like the mayhem around me so I lie down and close my eyes to shut out the din.

Ken comes over and sits beside me. Before the residential I was hoping to discuss some plans in the event of me having an episode, which is, I think, a very real possibility. Ken was meant to call me and didn't, and I feel the need to clear it with him.

'I don't trust you. You were supposed to call me and you didn't.'

'I'm sorry. I'm not good at calling people. I am good at holding spaces, though.'

I realise I have a choice. I could opt out, holding myself back, or I could trust Ken and let go. He is good at holding people through all kinds of difficult stuff. I really want someone to guide me through an episode if I have one and Ken is the only person I know who might be able to do that.

'OK.'

I raise my arms above my head, where they seem to want to go, dangling them behind me. My head tilts back a little to follow them. Ken puts his hand on my solar plexus. It feels like there's a force behind me trying to pull the energy out of my arms. Ken's hand is acting as an anchor and there's a subtle tug of war between us. It's like my arms are trying to get away while his hand is asking me to stay. An age seems to pass, and I've no idea what's happening with anyone else in the room. The music has played several tracks, but I'm focused only on this strange battle in my body.

When the music stops Ken takes his hand away and helps me sit up. Energy rushes back into my torso and I sob with a relief that the weird internal fight is over. I'm not sure if anybody won and I can't feel any sensation in my hands.

'I don't have my hands,' I say, aware of my odd way of expressing myself. Ken puts a blanket around me and rubs my hands to get the circulation going again.

I'm surprised to discover that most of the morning has passed and it's time to break for lunch. It's a strange atmosphere. We're all quite subdued and in our own space. Conversation seems forced and fake, utterly petty and pointless in contrast to what we've just been through.

After lunch the room is rearranged so that we students are lined up at one end while Ken and his assistants are at the other. In-between they've made a low wall of cushions. We're to take it in turns to get over the wall, which represents the obstacles in our life, to the other side where Becky will hand each of us a feather, a symbol of our taking up the challenge to face our fears. It sounds easy enough, a kind of psychodrama.

I wait in line and watch my fellow students make their way over, one by one. Each finds a different way, a unique strategy that reflects their personality. One smashes right through with great gusto. Another leaps over and we all cheer as if he's just won the Olympic hurdles. It's nearly my turn and I can feel a panic rising. Then I'm crying. What's wrong with me? I beckon Sean, the assistant, to pass me the box of tissues. I feel wobbly with fear. What am I afraid of? I walk towards the cushions with a calm exterior. I step over them and Becky hands me a blue feather. I take it nonchalantly, feigning an attitude of no big deal, my ridiculous coping strategy for life.

That night, I lie awake unable to get to sleep. The woman I'm sharing a room with is fast asleep. I don't know how people can crash out in strange places. I have trouble, especially if I'm with someone I don't know very well. At about 5am I give up, and sneak out quietly for a bath. The drops of water on the ceiling, created by the steam from the bath, drip down on me, and I get the feeling that God's around again. *Oh dear. That probably means another episode is on its way already.*

In the check-in circle in the morning, I let everybody know I didn't sleep a wink.

'Please be vigilant today. If I behave strangely then check with another student. If they think I'm behaving strangely then talk to Ken.'

'So the alarm is being raised,' Ken says before giving us our next set of instructions. We're going to have a truth circle. I seat myself next to Matt, feeling more part of the teachers and the assistants than the students. We're told to put our feathers in front of us facing to the left. As each person is ready, we're to speak our truth. Ken or Becky will assist us in turn, as they see fit.

I watch from the sidelines, wondering what they actually mean by truth anyway. One by one, people spout off some psychobabble about their mother or whatever and then go through some kind of process. Every so often Becky turns her feather in the opposite direction.

'Change feathers,' she calls and everyone copies. It's a ruse to get us all to go deeper and I'm not falling for it. I want to tell them that it's all a load of shit. Everyone is speaking from a distorted version of themselves about this wound or that trauma. It's not who they really are. Their truth is not really *the* truth. It's just a layer of crap to get through to get to the truth.

My truth right now is that we are all a part of God and everything else is a big drama created by the ego to keep us away from remembering this. I'm annoyed and it looks to me to be as much a part of building

Becky and Ken's egos as it is trying to break through the students'. It appears to be an unconscious game they've all entered into, as part of the student/teacher role each is playing.

As one of the students is talking, I don't hear what she's saying because my attention is drawn to a strange image in the carpet in front of her. The face of an indigenous South American has appeared. There's a big, black gap where his teeth should be and he's grinning manically, proudly displaying only one single tooth.

Now a different pupil is talking, but I can't concentrate on his words either because I see another image of a different head in the carpet in front of him. The face is covered in what looks like flesh-coloured latex. The nose is flattened so that the nostrils are widened and the bridge pointed. The eyes are closed in their sockets and the mouth is gaping open, writhing in pain.

Everyone has spoken except me. Ken and the others are waiting expectantly. It's my turn but I have nothing to say. I daren't speak what I'm thinking or experiencing. Perhaps I'm supposed to talk about some childhood event that I probably need to work through like everybody else.

I waffle on about a bad play review I got when I was nineteen. It's all I can think of to say. It's certainly not my truth but it might explain why I've now got stage fright.

'You're not in your body,' Ken says accusingly.

'I am,' I respond defensively.

'No. You're not in your body,' he repeats. I don't really know what he means. If I were out of my body, wouldn't I be looking down on myself from the ceiling or something?

'So how is it that I can feel my bottom is numb from sitting down so long?' Ken doesn't say anything. Instead Becky hands me a segment of lemon and tells me to suck on it. I put it between my lips and bite down on the yellow fruit. My eyes and face wince at the sourness and it feels like I'm receiving a punishment.

We break for dinner and some of the female students gather round me. One of them wants to try a piece of the lemon as if she's missing out. Like I got the special lemon treatment. *Is it just me or has everyone regressed to being children in the playground?*

After dinner we circle-up again, but I can't tell you exactly what happens. There's a gaping black hole in my memory. It's just a blank, like a drunk's blackout. I'm told later that Ken tries to bring me back.

'EMMA!' he shouts. 'EMMA! *COME BACK INTO YOUR BODY!*'

I'm slumped over and apparently look like I've checked out, like my body is there but I'm not. I've no idea that Ken is shouting at me even though I apparently look him right in the eyes.

'I don't believe this medical model view of your psychosis!' he yells or something along those lines. He's got quite worked up and Matt intervenes, taking him aside. Whatever he says does the trick because Ken reels himself in. Matt is one of Ciaran's best friends. They're both in the same men's group and I find out later that Matt thinks Ken and I are engaged in some kind of shamanic warfare. I don't know what that means but it puts a stop to the support I was hoping to receive from Ken.

I don't know if I sleep that night because again, I don't remember. I do recall walking into the main hall for the morning session though. There are mats all over the floor, which means we're finally doing some shiatsu.

I'm directed to Sean, the assistant. His futon is covered in crinkled creases that look like an aeroplane crash. They form a pointed dent at the top, crumpled wings and more wrinkles where the tail would have landed. The messy mattress doesn't give me any confidence in Sean but I lie down placing my head, arms, and legs in the crash zone.

Sean looks eager. His touch, though skilled and gentle, doesn't really make contact with me emotionally. I can feel him physically but I'm out of reach and he's not able to get to me. I can see that he wants to, but he's out of his depth. Or maybe I'm just too far away.

After my treatment, I'm taken outside to sit on the grass. Someone must have called Ciaran because he arrives and sits himself down next to me, crossing his long legs. He's still looking up at Ken and Matt, listening to them, not making any connection with me. His large black shiny pupils give away his fear. Maybe that's why he doesn't say hello, or make any show of affection towards me.

A flash of his childhood role, like a Polaroid camera delivering a photograph, comes to me. A sense of the little boy Ciaran gradually forms: his dad used to send him off on drug errands, a pawn to do his dirty work and now Ciaran's still playing that role, having to do Ken's for him. He doesn't appear to want to be here but is doing his duty anyway, because nobody else has been able to help.

Ken and Matt go back inside to continue with the activities for the day. Ciaran sits quietly next to me not making any conversation.

Gentle, feather-like rain drops from the sky and Ciaran picks me up in his arms as I clasp him around his neck. He walks us towards the shelter of a small tree, to protect my modesty. I've no idea that I've wet myself. As he does so, the world around us darkens like a solar eclipse, except for a beam of light that shines down onto Ciaran's face, like stage lighting: the heavens pointing to the hero of the hour.

I make it through a strange night with a witch and the devil to contend with. Ciaran sits with me while I writhe around in bed. When he goes off to take a break, one of the students covers for him. I don't know Pete very well. He doesn't say much in class. Ciaran knows him through his men's group.

Pete breathes deeply and slowly and loudly. I rotate ninety degrees, lying sideways with my head hanging over the edge and my hair dangling. I spit small blobs of saliva, watching them drip down strands of my matted hair.

I'm that witch from a long time ago.

Pete's eyes are tiny red slits, the devil keeping watch.

I feel calmer and more serene in the morning. It's the last day of the residential and I'm disappointed Ken wasn't able to do more. It doesn't seem to me like he did very much at all. So much for being good at holding spaces.

The air feels soft and warm for a May morning and Ciaran sits beside me on the bench at the end of the garden. He's arranged for the other students to come and see me, one at a time, to pay their respects and say farewell. I may have missed out on whatever grief process was going on yesterday but today I'm getting an honouring to make up for it and it's entirely Ciaran's doing.

Each student walks down the path reverently, exchanges a few words with me and gives me a hug. I feel like a queen while Ciaran, my king, remains quietly by my side, proudly watching on.

CHAPTER SIXTEEN

Homecare

I knew there was a high risk I would have another episode during the shiatsu residential. It's not the shiatsu itself that set me off. After all, we hadn't actually done any when I lost it. I'm pretty sure it was the intense and intrusive nature of the initiation process. I question the wisdom of digging around for psychological material that might not be ready to be integrated. It takes a certain strength and a readiness to be able to hold yourself through deep therapeutic work. Not everyone has developed that skill. People with certain vulnerabilities would probably do well to avoid it. My ego has shattered twice before so maybe it's too fragile for this kind of group work.

The ego is a sense of self we construct as part of the socialisation process we go through as children. We're not born with one but rather develop it over the first three years of our life. It doesn't actually exist as a physical thing. It's a construction of the mind, a set of beliefs about ourselves. Over time we associate more and more with this created personality, which helps us fit into society and be socially accepted. This in turns helps us survive. But it is a false identity we've constructed in order to get our needs met.

In a Western culture, the ego is encouraged to be individualistic, competitive, selfish, defensive, and ultimately separating. Different cultures sanction different qualities, through parenting, education, media, and law. A spiritual awakening can be seen as a process of becoming aware of who we really are, beneath all of this conditioning, our true selves. When my ego dissolves, like it does during my episodes, I become part of the collective consciousness, feeling oneness with all of life, no longer separate.

According to the psychological world, my goal is to strengthen my ego so that it doesn't disintegrate. I find it ironic that most people in the spiritual world are aiming for the opposite: to lessen the ego. It's great to feel liberated from the identification with it but it makes me realise why I need it—for self-preservation. And as long as my ego is intact, I can stay out of hospital. However, I haven't fully grasped the importance of that yet. I'm still allowing others to dictate the treatment I get, especially if they're responsible for looking after me, like Ciaran is.

Ciaran's got an advance to write a memoir so he works from home these days. An agent spotted him at a talk he was giving about his early life as an addict and criminal. She knew she could find a publisher for his story. We've put a desk in the corner of the living room where he taps away at the noisy keyboard. With him there, it means he can keep an eye on me so I can avoid another hospital admission.

I was up front with Ciaran about my episodes when we first met. I also told him about spiritual emergencies and how important it is to me for people in my life to be open to this perspective. He's quite a spiritual guy and with his background in shiatsu, which is not a mainstream approach to health, he's open-minded about alternative therapies. I'm grateful to be able to stay in my peaceful cottage while I go through another episode.

When he needs to go out, he calls on my friends to come and hang out with me, rather like a baby sitter. I spend most of my time in the garden, communing with nature, or listening to music in the back room. Ciaran's never very far away, especially when I'm having a bath, in case I think I can breathe under water, which has been known.

I feel intensely the tiniest of things that I wouldn't normally notice: the air on my face has different moods; every sound the house makes is an expression of its character; the birds chat with each other in a language I can almost understand.

As I soak in the bath, Ciaran brings me my clothes. He holds up my grey cotton Thai wrap- around fisherman's trousers, readying them for me to put on when I get out. Clasping each end of the waist ties, he rests the wide skirt-like trousers against his body. He looks like a cross between a Tibetan monk and a bishop. I like this Ciaran, soft and gentle and like a devotional servant. He's normally too wrapped-up in himself, his work, and his worries to pay much attention to me.

I step out of the bath and into a towel, sensing the energy radiating from him. It's as soft as cotton wool and I want to feel his skin against mine and make love, this aware and innocent.

'Don't.' Ciaran moves away. 'It would feel abusive.' I think it would feel better than ever but I respect his view and choose to leave it there.

A friend comes over for the evening, my climbing partner. We go every week to the indoor wall in a converted church in St Werburgh's. She's much older than I am, and a better climber, which means she can lead harder routes that I otherwise wouldn't be able to try. We talk a lot, about relationships mostly, in-between our climbs.

We don't talk much this evening though. I'm not in that mode and she's not here to socialise. I'm a little delicate and sensitive to stimuli but on the whole I'm feeling content in myself.

When I get up to go to the bathroom, an extreme sensation hits me in the stomach, crippling and causing me to slump onto the floor. It's like a panic attack but with a different emotion. I don't know what it is but I've felt it before, in my last episode, by the front door, when my dad was waiting to drive me back up north.

My friend rushes over and takes my hand in hers, stroking it towards her. The gentle caressing reverses the inward spiral, drawing out the horrible energy, which settles me.

She calls Ciaran who returns from his evening out. I'm OK though. The difficult moment has passed.

* * *

Ken and Becky recommend a psychotherapist who's used to working with people like me. I'm not sure how they see me and what this woman's particular expertise is but I want to sort myself out so I book a session with her.

She seems quite startled by me and says very little. She looks like she's trying to shield herself from me, as if I'm contagious. Maybe I'm coming across a little over the top. I don't really know. I describe to her what happens to me.

'There's something you can do that will help,' she says.

'Great! What is it?'

'Stop and focus on what your senses are experiencing. What can you see? Taste? Hear? Smell? Touch?'

'Is that it? That's all I have to do?' It sounds very simple. I can definitely do that. I can't wait to get home to try it out, which I do as soon as I arrive.

I stand squarely in the centre of the back room and put my attention on my five senses. I look around the room noting everything I can see: the table and chairs, the floorboards, the stereo, the mirror on the wall. I move on to what I can taste: just neutral saliva, no particular flavour of anything recognisable. *What about my ears?* I can hear the birds in the garden, the fridge humming, and my own breathing. *What can I smell?* Not much, but I breathe in deeply through my nostrils looking for a scent. *And touch? What can I feel?* The sleeve of my blue cotton top is noticeable against my skin along my forearms. The waistband of my jeans is pressed against my hips. My feet are enclosed in my walking shoes.

Is that it? Nothing is happening. I pull my focus back slightly and try to include all the senses at once. It's just a simple widening of my attention. I do it sometimes when someone is talking over me. I concentrate on what I'm saying at the same time as listening to what they're saying. So now I try it, in the same way, but with five things instead of only two.

Suddenly, a million thoughts slam into my head, all vying for my attention. It's like the scene in *The Matrix* where row upon row of guns slide dramatically into the white space surrounding Neo. My head has opened up, sucking up sentences like a vacuum cleaner. They're not coming from me. There are too many of them to separate them out individually.

What the fuck? This isn't helping me. My head feels like it's going to explode. How do I make it stop? I don't know what to do. I pick up the phone and dial the psychotherapist's number.

'You know I can't help you, don't you?'

What does she mean she can't help me? Is that because it's out of appointment time or she can't help me full stop?

'No, I don't know you can't help me! I wouldn't have called otherwise.' I put the phone down, muttering some vague thanks and a farewell. Then, just as quickly as they all arrived, the sentences are gone.

* * *

I have a wisdom tooth that's overgrown. *Over-occluded*, the dentist always says to the assistant as he's inspecting my teeth. Every dentist I go to wants to extract it, to make room for the one on the opposite side that doesn't have enough space to grow properly. Right now it feels huge, really big in my mouth. I run my tongue along my top row of teeth, reaching the edge of the last one, where it meets the others. It must be twice as big as its neighbours. It really ought to come out, I think. I've had two wisdom teeth out before and it was pretty straight-forward. I rotated my head around in synch with the dentist to help the process along. It feels ever so slightly loose, like it actually wants to come out. I could probably get it out myself if I tried. I fetch a claw hammer from the cupboard under the stairs and hook it into my mouth but there's no way it'll come out with this tool. Before I get a chance to remove it, Ciaran walks into the room. He panics, grabs the hammer and thrusts me against the wall with his hand around my throat.

'What are you doing?' he yells.

'It's OK. I was just trying to take my tooth out.' But it's hard to speak with his hand around my neck.

'With a claw hammer?' It does seem ridiculous and I don't really know how to make it sound less so.

'I can't leave you for five minutes.'

'I realised immediately it wasn't going to work. I wasn't really going to take my tooth out with it.' He loosens his grip then lets me go. But Ciaran's had enough and he's putting his shoes on and getting the car keys, readying himself to go.

'Come on. I can't do this any more. We're going to the hospital.'

Growing up surrounded by an ever-present danger has made Ciaran hypervigilant, and I think he's overreacting. But it's clear he's reached the end of his ability to support me. When I made a care plan, a document that outlines what I want to happen when I can't make decisions for myself, I made it clear that if Ciaran couldn't take care of me at home then I would go into hospital. The whole thing hinges on him being able to supervise me and if he can't do that for any reason, my plan becomes null and void.

At A&E a sweet young psychiatric member of staff deals with us. Ciaran tells him about the incident and I attempt to plea my case.

'I wasn't going to go through with it. As soon as I tried I knew it wouldn't work,' I say, trying to make it sound less crazy.

'I can't take care of her any more.' Ciaran looks across at me with tears in his eyes. His chin scrunches up and wobbles.

'I'm so sorry, Emma,' he says, as he's having me admitted. 'It's breaking my heart.'

'I know. It's OK. I'll go.'

There's no more questioning about how I am and what I need. They turn their attention to finding me a bed.

'While I'm here, I've got a mole I'm a little worried about,' I say to the young doctor, changing the subject. A large brown splodge on my thigh looks to me like it might have got bigger. 'I wouldn't normally bother someone about it, but as I'm here.'

'Just give it a name and keep an eye on it.' I sense the doctor's not taking me too seriously. He doesn't even look at it.

The reframing of my psychosis as spiritual emergency doesn't make any difference to the care I get. Nobody is able to guide me through. They mean well and believe in what they're doing. Ciaran resorts to the same old psychiatric model to have me admitted. I'm not going into hospital because of my need; I'm going because of his. And that's me all over.

CHAPTER SEVENTEEN

Fight

As usual, most patients on the psychiatric ward spend all day in the living room watching telly and chain-smoking. I've got my own room with familiar standard issue nasty carpets and basic furniture. It's like a prison cell, minus the toilet, but at least I can get away from the zombies and cigarette smoke. For something to do in the evenings, I soak in the bath with lavender essential oil that I brought with me. It also helps me sleep.

I wake in the pitch black of night. That horrible feeling is gnawing at my stomach again. I make myself as small as possible, wrapping my arms around my knees. I want to scrunch up so tight I could compress all the space out of me. I need to disappear into a black hole. I tighten up even smaller and crawl under the bed to get into the darkest corner. The hard synthetic carpet rubs my knees until they're red.

Ciaran visits and we take a walk around the grounds. I stop at the rose garden and close my eyes to take in the rich scent of one of the flowers. There are so many layers to the odour: vanilla ice cream followed by a hint of peach and then at the bottom of it some candy floss.

'It's like wine tasting. Which rose do you prefer by its smell?' Ciaran joins me but he's not really into it. He seems a little distracted.

'I like the peach one. It's amazing how different they all are.' He's still not responding so we walk on past the hospital chapel and sit under a willow tree for some shade. Ciaran's fair skin can't withstand this heatwave.

'Are you coming again tomorrow?' I ask hopefully.

'I don't know,' Ciaran replies. 'I'm here now.'

'What does that mean?' I feel a little hurt.

'I can't make any promises. I'm taking it one day at a time.' Fear creeps into my belly. I want assurances and guarantees.

There's a guy on the ward called Gabriel with long, grey, wiry, matted hair who's always accompanied by two male members of staff. It's touching to see them, one on either side of him, like a band of brothers, protecting him from himself. As I'm heading back to my room, he shuffles down the corridor towards me, his two bodyguards either side. When he sees me he stops, drops his jaw and his eyes widen like he's seen an angel or something. He pauses for a moment, stupefied, then he turns around and bends over, dropping his pyjama bottoms. I'm sure it's not an insult to me but more a demonstration of his self worth. His two sidekicks tug on the cotton drawstring of his PJs, pulling them up to recover his decency. I reach for the door handle to my room, leaving them fussing in the corridor.

My parents visit, too. They bring with them an air of being on holiday even though they're covering for Ciaran while he's away for the weekend. They speak to someone who lets them take me out for the afternoon. We spend an interminable amount of time in the car, driving through Bristol, down all the back streets. Mum and Dad are keen to see where the office that I've just started working at is.

I've been doing a lot of temping in-between directing contracts, which are now few and far between. The organisation I'm working for has created an alternative educational curriculum for kids who don't do well at school. The job is dull but the place seems like it's trying to do a good thing for young people who don't fit into the system. I liked the induction I went through, finding out about the organisation and the great work it is going. They seem to have innovative methods and at one point showed us a video of a ball beings passed around. We were told to count how many passes it made. Nobody saw the man in a gorilla suit walk through the room and we didn't believe one had done so until they played back the clip. What does that tell you about how selective our attention is, and how little we see of the reality around us?

We drive past the offices and then carry onto Dyrham Park, which is over an hour away. I have little interest in visiting stately homes but my parents are National Trust members.

I'm feeling very wobbly from being in the car too long. It's ungrounding travelling over land at an unnatural speed, in a metal box, catapulting my body forwards while my energy doesn't have time to catch up. When I get out, I feel like I've just stepped off a boat, still bobbing up and down. I slam the door shut, passive-aggressively. My dad has obviously not taken any notice of my care plan. It states clearly that long car journeys are not advised. He's probably not even read it. I've been honing it ever since the second episode when the social worker came to visit. I thought it wise to update it before the shiatsu residential.

When we walk into the busy tearoom, lots of heads turn to look at me. I feel uncomfortable and exposed. Crowds of people is another thing on my list of things to avoid. The clatter of cups, bashing out of the coffee grounds, tinkling of teaspoons on ceramic saucers feels like too many noises all at once.

'People are looking at me.'

'They're probably just thinking how beautiful you are.' Mum tries to make me feel better but it's too intense. I can't stay. This whole thing was a bad idea.

She links her arm through mine and walks me back to the car.

* * *

After my usual three weeks in hospital I'm discharged, to pick up the pieces of my life once again. A letter arrives from Ken saying that since I didn't complete the residential, which he sees as a course requirement, I'm unable to graduate. I'm livid. It's the only shiatsu school in the country that has a residential as part of the course. Missing two days of it is hardly a reflection of my abilities as a practitioner. We're only required to complete eighty per cent attendance on the course anyway so this is just a made-up excuse for Ken to fail me. The more I think about it the more hurt I am. Why does he want to fail me?

I get online and read about mental health discrimination law then call the Disability Rights Commission for advice. I write a letter responding to Ken's, outlining my position. I make a case for him having to make 'reasonable adjustments' for me on account of my mental health problems, that is, disability, and threaten legal action if he doesn't comply. I'm not going down without a fight.

Ken responds questioning whether I would be considered, in the eyes of the law, to have a disability. The bastard is using my own innocence against me. If he doesn't think my mental health is a disability then why does he want to fail me? I'm tormented and see no way through. Fighting him isn't working so I make an appointment to see him and Ciaran comes along to give me some moral support.

I sit in the usual client's chair with Ken in his usual practitioner one. Ciaran places himself to the side, forming a loose triangle.

'I don't want to fight with you, Ken. I've decided not to go down the legal route. If you don't want me to graduate then I'll have to accept that. I'm letting it go.' I pause, looking him directly in the eyes and feeling a little sad. 'There is something I'd like to say, though.'

'Yes. What is it?'

'When I expressed my concerns at the beginning of the residential, you claimed to be good at holding spaces. I think that was arrogant of you.'

'I don't think I was being arrogant. I was just expecting the best in the situation.'

It was his arrogance that was assuming the best, I think, but I leave it there. I didn't come to argue.

'I've decided to find another way for you to complete the course,' Ken continues. 'Would you be willing to have some one-to-one tutorials as an alternative to finishing the residential?' He's making the reasonable adjustments I requested.

I look over at Ciaran who's smiling.

'I'm so proud of you,' he says when we get home.

* * *

On a blustery Sunday the following January, Ciaran and I are out for a walk in the Mendips, with runny noses and pockets full of tissues. Ever since I could walk, our family put on walking boots every Sunday and drove into the countryside for a hike. I'm so glad I've found someone who likes walking too.

Halfway over a stile, I call him back to kiss him and to tell I love him. We're about the same height with me standing on the wooden step. But before I can say anything, he beats me to it.

'With the sun on your back and wind in your hair and snot in your nose and love in your heart, will you marry me?' he asks.

Fear jabs me in the guts. I couldn't be in a more appropriate place: I'm quite literally sitting on the fence. He's waiting for an answer, but I don't know what to say.

'Yes!' I default, without paying too much attention to my resistance. If it doesn't work out, we can always get divorced.

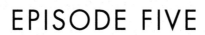

EPISODE FIVE

CHAPTER EIGHTEEN

Transition

The door seems to have closed on TV work. I went to an interview for a reality show where couples were to design and build their dream home. Each week a couple would get voted off and the last couple standing got to keep the house. I had already worked on a reality dating show and when one of the contestants was rejected, she had a nervous breakdown so I mentioned this in the interview.

'What safeguards do you have in place so that this doesn't happen on your show?'

'Well, there'll be psychologists making sure that we don't have any-body like that on the programme.'

Anybody like that? I don't like what he's implying. How do you ever know you're somebody 'like that' until you're publicly rejected on live television? I think we all have our limits and there's not people 'like that' and people who don't break down. We're all vulnerable given enough of a push.

'I'm trying to de-stress my life and the schedule sounds too gruelling for me at this time. Thanks for inviting me to this meeting with you but I don't think it's right for me.'

The door hasn't so much closed as I've slammed it shut.

After a year of going through the motions, exploring places in Dorset that Ciaran was interested in moving to, we've finally settled on Devon. Ciaran wasn't keen on Totnes at first but the whole Transition Town thing changed his mind. Transition is a grass roots, eco community movement that's been going viral since Transition Town Totnes first launched in 2006. One of Ciaran's friends from his men's group is involved and Ciaran was so impressed with the concept that it made him want to move here. I've wanted to move to Totnes since the qigong camp nearly four years ago. Lots of people on the camp lived here and when I asked David, my qigong teacher, where he lived, something weird happened in my body when he said Totnes, like I recognised the place even though I'd never heard of it. There's quite an alternative scene and it's twinned with Narnia. At least that's what people keep graffitiing on the 'Welcome to Totnes' sign. I need to be in a place where it's normal to be spiritual so I can strengthen that part of myself.

I've managed to get a job very quickly, doing exactly the same thing I was doing in Bristol. I'm a compliance officer for a healthcare recruitment company, making sure the applicants are legally and professionally qualified to temp. The place I work at has got a brand new computer system that the boss seems extremely proud of.

'It's taken the hunt out of the job,' I tell him. The software does all the work for you so it's mind numbingly dull. In Bristol, without this snazzy software, I made the job more fun by making a note of the applicants who only needed one more document in order to be ready to be put on a shift. I wrote their name on a whiteboard and when the post came in made sure to check it, giving a little cheer if a new temp had completed the process. Doing this kind of admin is boring enough but now my brain isn't needed at all, the rust rot has already set in after only three weeks. I don't imagine there'll be any filming work in Totnes and I can't face a lifetime of this.

'You're so miserable,' Ciaran says accusingly when I get home.

'Thanks for your support.'

'I'm just saying.'

'No, you said it like I was wrong for feeling miserable.'

'We've only just got here and you could at least be happy about it.'

'I'm doing the same crappy job I did in Bristol and it's killing me. I can't stand it.' Why can't Ciaran understand the despair I feel? For the last year I've been doing the same mind-numbing job and I've been struggling to remain positive.

'GET OUT!' Ciaran suddenly flips. I've never seen Ciaran change so suddenly. He's not the most stable person at the best of times but he normally has me to prop him up. Now I'm in the doldrums, it's threatening him on a very deep level. I understand but it doesn't make it any easier to be on the receiving end of. I try to walk across the room to get my bag but he blocks the way, squaring up to me, a wall I'm not allowed to pass.

'I SAID *GET OUT!*'

'I'm just getting my bag.'

'DON'T GET ANYTHING!' I duck and grab my handbag with the car keys in. I pull out of the driveway in shock and panic and don't know where to go. I head for the main road on autopilot, my belly quivering. I pull into a lay-by and reach for my mobile to call Ella. Ella from my first episode. We're not close friends any more but she moved down this way not long ago and I don't really know anyone else yet.

'I'm really sorry, Emma, but I've got three kids and I'm on my own a lot, so I've got hands full. I struggle at the best of times. I'm sorry, I just don't have the resources to help you.'

What the fuck am I going to do? All the other people I know down here are Ciaran's friends. With no other option I call Joe from Ciaran's men's group, the one who is involved with the Transition movement that inspired Ciaran to move here. His partner, Sarah, answers.

'Hi Sarah. I'm in a bit of a mess,' I say trying to choke back the tears. 'Ciaran's thrown me out and I've got nowhere to go.'

'Where are you?'

'I'm just sitting in the car near my house.'

'Why don't you come here? You're welcome to stay as long as you like.'

'Thanks Sarah. I'll be there in a few minutes.'

I don't really want to talk about Ciaran to his friends so I don't give them any details of the situation. They're both very sweet and welcoming and Sarah makes me a cup of tea. She shows me around their tiny garden that, in a short space of time, she's managed to fill to the brim with flowers and vegetables.

Over dinner Joe talks about the latest news from the world of Transition. He's actually co-founder of the Transition Network, which supports other communities to set up their own Transition Town wherever they are in the world.

'We've managed to get some funding to make a film.'

'You do know I'm a filmmaker, don't you, Joe?'

'I'd forgotten, actually. So how would you go about making a movie about Transition?' Joe smiles.

'Well it needs to have a story—so I would focus on finding a compelling narrative that would run through it.'

'If I gave you £15,000, what would you do with it?'

'I'd probably spend £10,000 on kit, which I would sell at the end of the production.'

'I like the way you're talking about it. You're saying the most intelligent things I've heard so far. Why don't you come in and have a meeting with us?'

'OK.' I'm excited now. This is just what I need to save me from the other job.

I don't want to outstay my welcome, though, so I only stay one night and then head to Bristol. My old housemate, Jane, has a spare room in her flat and is happy for me to crash there as long as I need. I feel more comfortable staying with her plus I can tell her everything that's happened.

'I give Ciaran so much emotional support and at the first sign of me struggling he freaks out.'

'What are you going to do?' Jane says, not colluding with me.

'I don't know.'

'Have you spoken to Ciaran?'

'I'm leaving it up to him to get in touch. He's the one who threw me out, remember?'

Jane sees right through my pain and gives me a look that tells me not to keep a score.

'And what will you do about the job?' She asks, changing the subject.

'I'm gonna quit. I'll ring them in the morning and tell them I'm not going back. I hate it.'

I put off calling Ciaran until I've softened.

'It's me.'

'Where are you?'

'I'm staying at Jane's.'

'Are you coming back?'

'I don't know.'

There's a pause.

'I can't afford to. I quit my job.'

There's another pause.

'What are you going to do?'

'I'll probably do some WWOOFing.'

'What's that?' Ciaran asks.

'Willing Workers On Organic Farms. There's a few places around Totnes that take people in.'

'Does that mean we won't be living together?'

'You haven't even said if you want me back.'

'Of course I want you to come back.'

'I can't pay my way.' I pause, hoping he'll offer to cover my share but he's not forthcoming.

'Would you be willing to pay my share of the rent until I've sorted something out?'

'OK.'

'OK. I'll be home tomorrow.'

* * *

I'm pleasantly surprised by the big, green ribbon Ciaran has put on our pale blue Ford Focus. It lets me know I'm not doing *everything* to prepare for our wedding. Dad sits in the front with Ciaran and Mum takes the back seat with me.

'Working class style,' Dad says to Ciaran.

'What do you mean?'

'Men in the front and women in the back.'

'What's middle class?' Ciaran asks in his soft west London tone.

'Couples together.'

Totnes Registry Office is not far from our little annexe flat in Dartington. I haven't put much effort into this part of the weekend. It's just the legal bit but we've managed to get it to fall on the 08/08/08. I'm wearing a blue Chinese silk skirt and bodice that I made years ago. There are no other guests apart from Ciaran's step-mum, who's one of the witnesses, plus her husband. Rose was much more of a mother to Ciaran, taking care of him when his dad was in prison. She was the sane and gentle constant who stuck by him even after she split with Ciaran's father.

The registrar loves his job. You wouldn't be able to tell that marrying people was an everyday thing for him. He manages to lead the ceremony with reverence even though we've not asked for anything special. It's very laid back and I feel totally at ease, no wedding nerves or second thoughts.

I sit in the only chair as we sign the register, tenderly stroking Ciaran's back, like a mother instinctively calming her child. The only thing I've requested is a piece of music: Eva Cassidy's *Fields of Gold*. The song is about commitment: about a man who has broken promises before, but is determined to make this relationship last. I'm well aware that Sting, who wrote the song, is Mum's favourite. Ciaran and Mum are both weeping but I feel serene and flooded with peace.

Rose and her husband don't join us for lunch at the White Hart on the Dartington Estate. I let them give us the space they think we want. We haven't booked anything, just going with the flow. After a gourmet burger and chips, we're serenaded around the grounds by impromptu musical accompaniments. It's the Dartington Summer School where world-class musicians teach master classes and people from all over the globe come together to train and perform. Elaborate Baroque pieces escape from windows and we stumble upon madrigals that float through the gardens. And the gardens are stunning. There are sculptures and immaculately kept borders, closely mown lawns and wishing well ponds. It would cost a fortune to get married here.

The rest of the afternoon is not so relaxing. There's lots of ferrying to and from Hazelwood House in preparation for our Sacred Wedding Weekend. It's only twenty minutes' drive but the roads are narrow and bendy with high hedges so you can't see around the corners. Dad is driving and the cake is perched on the back shelf. I sit in the back, focused on its safety. Ciaran's seated up front talking to Dad about his book, which has just been published. He loves to tell my parents about his work because they give him the praise he's looking for. They're both oblivious to the real task in hand, which is to get the cake safely to the venue. I'm trying not to be Bridezilla so I don't say anything about Dad's erratic and speedy driving. When a lorry suddenly appears around the corner, Dad slams on the brakes. The cake jolts forwards hitting my headrest, which luckily prevents it from flying across the car.

'THE CAKE!' I scream. '*AM I THE ONLY ONE WHO GIVES A SHIT ABOUT THE CAKE?*' They both look round to check the damage. 'It's OK. There's only a small dent in the icing.'

That evening, we have staggered hen and stag dos. First the women gather round a big fire outside to bless me with words of wisdom. The married ones talk about how hard marriage is. A shiatsu friend of Ciaran's, Laura, with her young daughter by her side, tells us how her relationship is the biggest challenge in her life. They're not telling me anything I don't already know but I'm glad they're not pretending that it's all a happy-ever-after fairytale. When we finish, the men have their turn at the fire pit.

At bedtime neither Ciaran nor I can get to sleep. I'm not worried about it because I'm not sure anyone sleeps the night before their wedding do they? The morning is a mixture of stress and bliss. We were hoping to have our ceremony outside but it's raining hard so I ask my friends to decorate the chapel with wild picked foliage. I tried to grow my own flowers, marigolds for an Indian feel, but I planted them too late so they didn't bloom in time.

My sister gives me a manicure and we talk about our grandmothers. Sally tells me about a psychic reading she had recently.

'The medium was absolutely spot on. She said, "You were out for dinner recently and all the cutlery was lined up and you didn't know which to use." And we *were*. We went out to this really posh restaurant and I was really stressed because I didn't know which spoon to use for the soup. Then the psychic said, "You suddenly knew to pick up the one on the far right. Well, that was your grandmother guiding you. She often comes to help you."'

I rarely spend any one-to-one time with my sister. We don't have much in common. We played together as children but our teenager years saw us grow apart. One of my earliest memories is with Sally, in Nigeria. We had put our dolls in the tree in the garden before heading out in the car somewhere with Mum. When we got back, as we came up the driveway, we laughed our heads off to discover they were still there, where we had left them. I was tickled by the idea that the physical world was a constant thing that had continuity, even though I wasn't there to uphold it. I vividly recall the cosmic ridiculousness I felt without having the words to communicate it. I'm not sure if my sister was amused for the same reason but it made her giggle just as much. There was a time when I would have laughed at the psychic medium story she's just told me, thinking her gullible. But now it's good to know I'm not the only one who thinks our grandmother might be guiding us.

It's only a couple of minutes' walk to the chapel from the house but it's absolutely throwing it down, so Dad drives us there. When he shows up at the door to collect me, I reach for the skirt of my dress but the loop to thread my finger through is dangling off.

'*Shit*. I need to sew it back on but I don't have time.'

'You're the bride, Emma. They can't start without you. Take all the time you need.' It only takes a couple of minutes and then we rush into the car trying to avoid the downpour.

'Ding-dong, ding-dong. Ding-dong, ding-dong. Ding-dong, ding-dong.' Dad mimics the wedding bells as he steers us down the gravel lane. One of Ciaran's friends is peering out of the front door and when he sees us arriving, goes back inside. He must be the lookout. There's probably someone at every wedding that has to wait at the door to give the nod that the bride has arrived. I haven't thought about this before. I quietly appreciate how other people are helping to pull this thing together, doing things I haven't thought of. I can almost let go of all the responsibility I'm holding.

Then the drumming starts. That's Ciaran's cue. The beat sounds tinny from outside the building, the acoustics unable to handle a *djembe*. I'm suddenly very nervous. There's a slight pause before Ciaran's opera-singing friend begins. His high warbling is totally unexpected. We've never heard him sing and had no idea he was a counter-tenor. I'm thoroughly confused and can't make out the song. It's supposed to be *This Little Light of Mine* but I don't recognise his version of it. My heart is thumping. I adjust my ears to listen better. I hear something about a long road and surrender to the words.

It has been a very long road to get to this point. It's been rocky with Ciaran, and I was never sure if we would make it this far. At thirty-eight years old, it's probably quite late in life to be getting married.

I give the signal to my nieces, my bridesmaids, and they walk into the main chapel, before Dad and I follow closely behind them. Emotion wells up inside me and I want to wail but fear squeezes it back down. My face contorts with the most excruciating battle between despair and terror and I don't want people to see me looking like this.

Finally I recognise the lyrics, which encourages me down the aisle. I've spent two months making this wedding dress, and familiar faces look suitably delighted. An old friend from Hong Kong smiles and I scan the room making sure I take it all in. It's not a big space so it's packed out and some people are standing. My Bristol friends are all on one row and my shiatsu friends sit together on another. My family are right at the front and my older brother is welling up. Ciaran is waiting next to the interfaith minister and he's beaming. When we get to the altar, Dad makes an exaggerated gesture of handing me over to Ciaran. I well up at the drama of losing a father, which is of course entirely imaginary. Once my grand entrance is over I relax a little and clock the emergency exit just behind the altar. If there were no such thing as divorce, I probably wouldn't be going through with this wedding.

Ciaran weeps as we say our vows and wipes the moisture from his face before we kiss, man and wife. The place erupts.

My next worry is Dad's speech, but he throws away what he's pre-pared and, inspired by the intimate and authentic feel of the occasion, decides to speak from his heart. He gets called Malcolm Obama for his oratory skills, in stark contrast to the best man, who crosses way over the line. He uses the occasion as a platform to campaign for the awareness of sex addiction. He actually thinks it's funny to compliment Ciaran's ability to pull *real* women as opposed to his own inferior internet porn habit. It's totally inappropriate, as there are quite a few children in the room. I have a horrified look on my face.

'It's all part of it,' someone mouths over to me. I just hope the kids have lost interest because he's been going on for so long.

The window behind us slams open and then closes but only my sister notices, convinced that Ciaran's dearly departed father is watch-ing over us.

Honeymoon

I don't sleep after the party. Ciaran has trouble too, complaining about the snoring he can hear through the walls. The next morning I feel quite wobbly. It's not from a hangover. Ciaran's a recovering addict so the reception was not your usual piss up. We only provided a bar at the last minute, when a few people objected to our plans for a dry wedding. No, I'm delicate and emotional because of the lack of sleep. I don't feel right so we decide not to go too far afield for our honeymoon. I don't really want to go anywhere but Ciaran seems set on at least making it to North Devon.

He makes a few calls from his mobile, trying to get hold of some sleeping tablets for me. There's little open on a Sunday but Ciaran wheels and deals his way around the system. His previous skills as a drug addict are coming in handy, as is his new status as a husband, to cut through the bureaucracy. He manages to arrange a prescription we have to collect from a large pharmacy on the edge of Torquay. I wait patiently in the car, feeling 100 per cent the burden that Ciaran is making me out to be.

En route to Appledore, we stop at a regional BBC office in Barnstaple. Ciaran's been invited onto the Jeremy Vine show and I insist he does it, even though promoting his book is work and we're supposed to be on our honeymoon. I don't mind waiting in the car park and tuning in live. It's quite exciting. I can't bear Jeremy's shock jock style but he's away on holiday so there's a stand-in. The interview is transmitted down the line, making it seem like Ciaran's in the studio with the presenter in London.

'Was it difficult to write about?'

'Absolutely. But there's a saying, no tears in the writer, no tears in the reader.'

I listen proudly, choked up by his story. It gets me every time.

Ciaran exits the building and strides across the car park towards me.

'Were you listening?'

'Of course I was! You were brilliant.'

'Really?' His face lights up.

'I don't know how you do it. You sounded so calm.'

We eventually make it to Appledore, where there's a folk music festival. The owners of the B&B remind me of Ken and Becky. I get a weird feeling about them. Something about doppelgängers. I know they're not Ken and Becky but it feels like they are. I can't really explain it. It just feels odd.

We head to the music venue, which is just a boxy room with rows of plastic chairs. We seem to wait an age for the musicians to arrive. A black guy walks into the hall and stands out among the sea of otherwise white faces. My stomach tightens. I feel like I'm in a police line-up looking right at my abuser. I know it's not really him, but I'm all knotted up with fear. My armpits are prickling and my face is flushing with an uncomfortable emotion. I manage to sit through it, half-focusing on the music to distract myself.

The next morning I still haven't slept and Ciaran's getting irritated because my insomnia is interfering with his sleep. He's very tired but I feel wired and need to walk it off so we drive to the beach and put our walking boots on.

'Ciaran, I'm definitely into Amber now.' We have a traffic-light system to gauge how I am, as part of my relapse avoidance. Amber means I need to minimise any stresses and avoid long car journeys. I need to do grounding things like walking. If I don't, I'm in danger of going into the Red, which probably means hospital again.

'What shall we do?'

'Why don't you call James Abraham and see what he says?' I suggest.

The strong sea breeze carries Ciaran's voice away so he has to shout down his mobile. I lean in closer trying to catch James's response on the speakerphone.

'You have the evil eye on you.' Ciaran and I look at each other, pulling the same expression, as if to say, *This is bullshit.* 'Because of your wedding, there's jealousy projected onto you, and this energy is disturbing Emma.' Ciaran's never been that impressed by James, and I've always been in two minds. The evil eye! Who talks like that? It sounds like an Abraham blag. I wave my hand and shake my head, gesturing Ciaran to end the call.

Ciaran and I paid James a hundred quid to check out why my house wasn't selling, before we moved to Totnes. I had no idea there was a financial collapse about to take place and no one was buying. James used his pendulum and said that it was because there were malevolent entities in the house that were obstructing the sale. He then proceeded to speak in what sounded to me like a made-up language, and waved a big crystal wand around to get rid of them. Predictably, they were hiding in the corner cupboard upstairs before he apparently chased them out. His babbling words had me in stitches. I wanted to believe him but it was so utterly ridiculous I just couldn't take him seriously. I've had little faith in James since then, and this evil eye interpretation is the nail in the coffin now.

'I think we need to do a ritual to close the ceremonial space down,' I say when Ciaran catches me up.

'Right,' Ciaran says, pondering.

'The interfaith minister invited in the four directions, opening up a powerful portal, lit a candle to your father, and asked for support from spirit world but the celebrant didn't close any of it down afterwards. Let's do something on the beach, here.'

'Like what?'

'I don't know yet. Something will come to us.'

The tide is out revealing a wide expanse of beach: damp, compacted, reddish sand. Ciaran grabs a driftwood stick and draws a large circle on the copper coloured ground.

'Stand in the middle of this,' he instructs. I walk into the centre of the fine, etched line. He draws another one a few metres away and stands in it. 'You need to sever your circle and walk out of it and into mine,' he shouts above the wind.

'Sever?'

'Yes. Wipe out the line and walk through the gap.'

'"Sever" sounds a bit extreme and very masculine.'

'Well, what do you suggest?' he barks at me defensively.

'Something a little more feminine,' I say, ignoring his outburst. 'Let's draw a third circle in-between, overlapping these two and both step into it together.'

'OK,' he agrees and marks one out. Ciaran puts the stick down and takes a step into the new space, still in his own circle but now also in the linking one. 'As I step out of this circle,' he says commanding my attention, 'I am closing down the space we've opened up and thanking the spirits for working with us.' He takes another step over the boundary of his circle, now fully in the neutral one. I follow his lead making my own speech to the spirit world and cross over to join him.

'Now I need to go for a long hike around the coast to tire myself out.'

'I'm too tired. I don't think I have the energy,' Ciaran says, probably hoping I'll change my mind.

'Then I'll have to go on my own,' I say, feeling a little sad.

'But it's our honeymoon.'

'I'm not well, Ciaran, and if I carry on not sleeping I'll have another episode!'

Ciaran accompanies me to the start of the coast path. We check the map and make plans to meet in Clovelly, which looks like a good fifteen miles away.

There's a pavement of rocks jutting out along the shore. As we pick our way over them, dodging the small rock pools, a strange image comes to me. But this time it's from the future.

I'm a TV presenter, sitting on these very rocks giving a final piece to camera in an end-of-the-world broadcast. All the creatures of the seas are gone: no dolphins, no whales, no seahorses. A snapshot of the last moments on earth. But this won't be a seaside postcard that future generations will feel nostalgic about, because they won't exist. This is a prophetic image, a warning, like the ghost of the Christmas future. It leaves me wondering what would be the point of this vain media transmission, if there isn't anybody alive to watch it?

Ciaran and I say our goodbyes and I walk off alone.

I can see a settlement, far off in the distance, most likely Clovelly. But after walking a good few hours around the headland and into a large bay, it actually looks like it's getting further away. It's probably an optical illusion caused by the curve of the coastline. I feel disheartened and wonder whether I can walk the rest of the way. Fifteen miles is twice as far as I would normally go.

I stop at a junction to a path that turns away from the coast and heads inland. What shall I do? I sit under a tree and wait for some guidance. The ancient coastal woodland has been shaped by the wind. Farmland surrounds the forest with open pastures sloping up the side of the valley. There's no sign of any roads or buildings. I'm probably about halfway and it feels far enough.

I climb the stile onto the densely wooded path that turns away from the sea, and hope it meets the main road. Eventually I do hit an A road, at an old village primary school, which is now a dwelling. I call Ciaran and describe the place, giving this building as a landmark, so he can find me on the map. Ciaran tells me to wait and says he'll be right there.

He seems a little irritated when he arrives. He says there's a pub not far away where we can get some dinner. I didn't realise it was that time already. It's a good job I aborted my walk. The inn is busy with holiday-makers. People are looking at me, and one woman in particular keeps flashing glances my way.

We order and wait in silence. There's a disapproval in the air but I don't know what I'm supposed to have done wrong. The food arrives and I can't wait to finish eating and get out. I don't like feeling people's eyes on me and Ciaran has disappeared into his head.

'I'm really struggling, Ciaran. I need to go home.'

We pay the bill and leave.

The drive home is long and dark. It's like we're moving through a vacuum at the end of the world and the movement forwards is simply an illusion. We're really just standing still, on the same spot, as time and space rush past the windows while the view through the windscreen stays the same: blackness, white lines, headlights, and road.

Back at the flat. Ciaran's pissed off about having to come home, and I'm pissed off that we went in the first place. This is not a good start to our marriage. We climb into bed, leaving our unpacking for tomorrow.

At 1am I notice the clock, but I'm not sure if I've been to sleep. I've got that horrible feeling of impending death again. Annihilation is coming to get me. The feeling that marks the official start of my episodes.

With Ciaran asleep beside me, I think about his father committing suicide.

It must have taken a lot of courage to actually go through with it: to know you're going to die and still choose it. I couldn't do it. I don't want to die. I'm terrified. I want someone to help me. I can't do this alone.

I get out of bed, careful not to disturb Ciaran. I pick up the phone and dial 999.

'Hello. Police, ambulance or fire?'

'Er, hello. I'm not sure. I want help to die.' Saying it out loud makes it sound like I want to kill myself but that's not what I mean.

'We don't help people take lives, madam. We only help save them.' The man sounds jaded. And he sounds exactly like Ciaran's best man, the one who made that long, inappropriate speech. But it can't be him. This isn't his job. He asks me for some details, my name and address and then I hang up and head back to bed.

At about 2am there's a loud, purposeful knock at the door, which wakes Ciaran.

'Who the fuck is that?' he mutters.

Neither of us goes to the door, hoping that whoever it is will go away. Next we hear rustling and heavy boots on the carpet stomping through our small flat. The bedroom door opens and two men walk in, dressed in wildlife ranger-green uniforms.

'Did somebody call for an ambulance?'

Ciaran looks at me questioningly.

'I dialled 999.'

'For fuck's sake.' Ciaran turns to the paramedics who are still waiting at the door. 'I'm really sorry. My wife's having a psychotic episode. Everything's fine. Sorry to have wasted your time.'

'No trouble at all. If you're sure everything's OK, we'll be on our way.' And they leave. Ciaran turns over with an irritated sigh, pulling the duvet over his shoulders.

The next morning the atmosphere is tense. Ciaran and I are at each other's throats, and find ourselves on the verge of a terrifying physical confrontation—it is too much.

A couple of women from the Crisis Team arrive. Ciaran's called them and told them what's happened. They sit on the sofa and Ciaran's the first to speak.

'Emma's got to go. I can't handle this any more.'

'We're here for Emma, Ciaran. If you're finding it too difficult, you're the one who has to leave.'

It seems obvious when they put it like that. Last time he held me down, when I tried to pull my tooth out with a claw hammer, I went obediently into hospital because Ciaran couldn't handle it. The idea of him having to go instead of me is a revelation. Why hadn't I thought of that? I'm suddenly very grateful for the Crisis Team.

'Do you feel OK to be on your own, Emma?' I nod at the woman with the big scar in the middle of her chest.

'One of us will come to see you every day to make sure everything's OK. OK?'

'Thank you,' I say, wanting to cry.

My friend Sonja comes around to support me. Nearly everyone I know down here in Totnes is a therapist, and Sonja is no exception. We go out for a walk on the Dartington Estate. She takes me to an area of woodland she regularly goes to, stopping to let the trees know we're entering before stepping over the barbed wire fence. It's totally normal down here to talk to nature spirits.

I've not known Sonja very long. She's in the woman's group I set up that meets fortnightly. She works for the Transition Network and is passionate about inner transition: the idea that if we want to change the world out there then first we have to understand and change our inner world because that's what creates the outer. She's a great asset to the women's group and when we met up before my wedding she noticed and pointed out that I was holding far too much. She encouraged me to delegate more, to hand responsibility over to others. I appreciated her suggestion and she's just the person I need right now to help me.

The other side of the wood leads to a field where Sonja suggests we sit down.

'Close your eyes and notice your breath, whether it is shallow or deep.'

Listening to her instructions makes me realise how much I'm in my head.

'I can feel a strange chaotic ball of energy here.' I scoop the air just above the top right hand side of my head. 'It's like I need to stroke it.'

'Then stroke it,' Sonja encourages me gently. Her trust in me makes me trust my sense too. I brush the air above me without touching my head. Short, slow movements; within seconds the wire wool feeling is gone.

We continue on like this for a good twenty minutes and, bit by bit, I iron myself out, uncrumpling all the creases inside.

'Thank you,' I say at the end.

'I didn't really do anything.' She seems disappointed by her contribution.

'Yes, but I wouldn't have thought to do it without your prompting.'

Mia Carter, from the Crisis Team, visits me again. She's friendly and treats me like a normal human being. I like the way she makes no attempt to hide the huge scar down the middle of her chest where she must have had heart surgery. It makes her seem more human. And it was Mia who put Ciaran straight about who had to go.

'I don't like the label "psychosis",' I tell her.

'What would you prefer me to call it?'

'A spiritual emergency. It's when a person has an awakening that's ...'

'Spiritual emergency. Yes, I've heard of that,' Mia says. I feel like Daf-fyd Thomas from *Little Britain*'s 'Only Gay in the Village' sketch. I think they must be quite progressive down here. That's probably why she doesn't talk down to me.

I manage to stay out of hospital and Ciaran comes back home after a couple of days.

'I was really angry that you didn't take any notice of my care plan. We shouldn't have gone away after the wedding when I wasn't sleeping.'

'But it was only meant to be an hour away.'

'It took us hours to get there, and having to deal with strangers and unfamiliar places was too much for me to cope with.'

Ciaran goes quiet.

'I just wanted us to have a nice honeymoon.'

'I know. We'll go somewhere next year instead.'

CHAPTER TWENTY

Premiere

This most recent episode is the most 'successful' one to date. Perhaps it was just a minor one but I like to think it was recognising I was in Amber and insisting on going home early from our honeymoon that avoided precipitating me into the Red zone. Being in a rural setting was conducive to recovery, with nothing to overstimulate me. I also had support from people who were open-minded about spirituality. I stayed out of hospital because the Crisis Team did a great job of advocating for me.

When Ciaran told the ambulance men that I was having a psychotic episode, I felt betrayed. His use of the old language showed he has no real faith in my spiritual perspective. The man I hoped would take care of me in sickness and in health is not able to do so. I don't blame him. His own traumatic childhood has left an indelible mark that means he needs emotional support most of the time.

Anyway, I'm back in action now, in time to start on the Transition film. They want to make a documentary to inspire others in the world to set up Transition. I'm co-directing it with a guy called Nick Jones from a production company in Totnes. He's quite old school and a little jaded.

'How's growing a carrot going to change the world?'

He's got a point, but it's the feeling of the movement that I'm struck by.

When I was in Bristol, I walked around the city feeling quite angry about how everybody was seemingly oblivious to the effects of our modern lifestyle. I hated going into supermarkets with everything packaged, imported, and out of season. The fridges don't have doors because they think people will buy less so it's not only freezing cold, it's a massive waste of energy.

Totnes seems more progressive. The fact that so many people have come together to create Transition means that people actually believe they *can* change things. They're not waiting for governments to do anything and are just getting on with it themselves. I like being among that. It makes me realise how powerless I felt before.

When I moved down here I thought that would be the end of my filming career. I was expecting to build my shiatsu practice instead, but every other person here is a therapist. The town is saturated with flyers for every kind of healing modality you can think of. It's a graveyard for practitioners. Being seen around filming various Transition Town Totnes projects is a good way to meet people. I'm suddenly that girl with the camera, and I feel very lucky to be the person making this film. It's an opportunity I so desperately needed.

*   *   *

I'd always imagined I would go to Bali for my honeymoon: romantic evenings making love in the sea; sleeping in a beach hut with tropical fruits for breakfast; exploring the ancient spiritual ways of the Balinese people. But money is tight, so we've come to North Devon again; the Hartland peninsular this time. We were going to walk along the coast path but the first day was so tiring, a constant challenge of ups and downs that irritated Ciaran, and we've given up on that.

We doze through the early morning sunrise, with the light making the pink lined tent quite psychedelic. I'm feeling sensuous from sleeping on the ground and breathing the fresh sea air. I feel the familiar pull to make love that ovulation brings. I want Ciaran to explore my whole body, stroking every contour with his hands and lips. But he never does and I never ask. *Maybe marrying him was a mistake*, I think.

I get up, avoiding looking at him and feeling that familiar sinking guilt for questioning whether we should be together or not. We head for the beach and I sit down, looking out at the sea. I really wanted to make love this morning and now we can barely talk to each other.

Ciaran heads off to make a phone call. He'll be speaking to one of his many recovering addict friends for some support. I throw a few rounded pebbles into the sea in a defeated gesture. Ciaran returns and tells me to close my eyes. I put my hands over them, my eyelashes flickering against my palms.

'OK. Now open them.'

In front of me is a huge heart shaped stone, the size of a football. We've been giving each other stones like this since the first time I hunted around for one on the beach in Cornwall. It was the weekend I went to the wedding and brought back the tulips whose vase he 'accidentally' smashed. That same weekend he slept with someone else.

Tears fill my eyes. Ciaran smiles like a little boy, his gesture silently pleading 'don't leave me'. I feel so much love for him but I also feel sad for myself. What can I do but smile back? And with my response, nothing is resolved.

* * *

The film premieres at the Transition Network Conference in London. Nick pulled out in the end and I ended up editing it without him. We had an ongoing argument about what software to use for the edit. He wanted to use a Rolls Royce of a system called Avid. But this would mean that in future the footage would only ever be accessible via their expensive-to-hire edit suite. I wanted to edit using Final Cut Pro so that all the rushes could be available to the Transition Network or anyone else who might need them at a later date.

'Are we having this same conversation again, Nick? I can't believe we're actually having this conversation again.' I was irritated. I don't like losing it in a work setting. It's not very professional so I decided to pull out and let Nick do it his way. If we couldn't agree on which system to use, it didn't really bode well for the rest of the edit. Luckily Nick was thinking exactly the same thing, and said it first, so I graciously accepted his 'resignation' instead of offering mine.

The hall is packed full with about 500 people who've all come to discuss Transition. I give a brief introduction describing the process of making the film.

'Because it's a community-led movement, I wanted to make a film that reflected that. And necessity is the mother of invention. We couldn't afford to fly around the world to film all the stories, and what with climate change wouldn't have wanted to anyway. So instead, I invited everyone to send in footage. I received about 100 hours and there was some real gold dust in it. So it's not only a film about the Transition community, it's also made *by* the community.'

The film gets a standing ovation but I can't take it in. I don't think it's *that* good. I think they're all really applauding the success of Transition itself.

Not long after this, someone forwards me an email from a local organisation who wants a promo for their website. They don't have much money but it gives me an opportunity to make an online video that I can use to promote myself. I manage to tick some boxes at the Job Centre, because of my mental health history, and get three hundred quid towards a camera. I find a second-hand Canon on eBay, an old eMac and some Final Cut Express software and go into business. Green Lane Films is born.

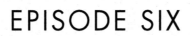

EPISODE SIX

CHAPTER TWENTY ONE

Shakti

Rachael waddles up the lane in a pair of wellies and a short skirt, innocently exposing her soft round knees. The curls around her face bounce in ringlets and her big brown eyes sparkle with life as she smiles. Ciaran's eyes are popping out of his head and I'm smiling on the inside. This is really going to test him!

We've moved into a big house just across the road that we can't afford. We had to leave the little annexe because the landlord and landlady are going to extend it. We wanted to stay in the same village so we've taken on a place that's far too big for us, renting out rooms we don't use as office spaces. Rachael is our first tenant. She's a singer-songwriter and has a contract with an online gaming magazine. Every week she composes and records a track, reviewing the latest video game, which she invariable dislikes. She's not into them at all. Her music makes more of a social comment on the gaming world than on the games themselves. Gaming addicts love her. She's their virtual fantasy girlfriend.

Rachael recommends my new filming business to a woman she knows. Isabella Navarro offers something called Shakti dancing, just for women. Apparently she wants to produce some DVDs so women can dance at home. It sounds straightforward enough. The filming opportunity doesn't pan out but I go along to the drop-in class anyway to see what it's all about. I wait until the first Thursday of the month, because that's when the website says that instruction will be given to newcomers. It turns out I'm the only one who hasn't been before, so Isabella decides to forgo the lesson, leaving me to follow along as best I can.

It's dark with the only light coming from a candle in the centre of the room. The other women seem to be focusing internally, swaying and floating their arms around. I don't like not knowing what I'm supposed to be doing so I just stretch out into the spaciousness of the music. I keep my eyes closed and notice all the tight places in my body, moving gently around them to tease them out of hiding.

'That's not the dance,' Isabella says to me afterwards. I feel a little crushed. How could I know the dance if she hasn't taught me? I compose an email asking to go to the next class for free. Isabella responds, acknowledging my anger and disappointment and leaves it up to me whether I pay or not. The next Shakti dance is on the winter solstice. There's an introduction for newcomers on the Friday evening and a whole day on the Saturday. I decide to just go for the lesson. A whole day might be too much for me. I don't want to have another episode.

Isabella has set up a projector that's playing footage of Indian women dancing with elephants from a film called *Ashes and Snow*. The slow motion accentuates their grace and power. What would it be to dance this sensuously? We're guided to close our eyes and relax. My face softens: my lips and lower lips too.

'There are no steps to learn. It's about reclaiming our true power as women. Uncoiling through layers of conditioning, from thousands of years of patriarchy and all the ways we've been silenced, to uncover the wisdom, our birthright that resides in our wombs.' Isabella has long, dark, wild and wavy hair. She wears thick black eyeliner and a finely netted skirt, a thoroughly modern witch.

The music is slow, with deep breaths, chiming bells, and whispers circling around the sound system. A female singer endlessly repeats the same phrase.

Re-turning. Re-turning. Re-turning. To the mother of us all.

'Find the gentle pulsing of your womb and move your hips around in a figure of eight. Let your arms be an expression of your heart.'

Grunts, groans, sobs, and gentle roaring can be heard from the women who have obviously danced before. Their noises penetrate my solar plexus where my energy feels paper-thin, setting off anxious jitters. I keep quiet. I haven't found my voice yet, or my womb for that matter.

At the end, I don't rush to leave. A woman sitting next to me strikes up a conversation. She's been dancing for a while and has been assisting Isabella with the class. Shelly has long, soft, curly hair and a gentleness in her voice but a sharpness in her eyes. I can't place her accent but she turns out to be from Israel via America. I end up talking about Ciaran.

'It took six months before he could hear that I wasn't enjoying myself in bed as much as he was.'

'What do you mean it took six months?'

'Well I told him three times over six months and it wasn't until the third time that he actually got it and properly heard me.'

'You told him three times on the first night?'

'No, over six months,' I correct her, thinking she hasn't understood me.

'So you didn't tell him three times on the first night?' Her voice is soothing and without judgement. The impact of it hits me, showing me the problem from a totally different perspective. Why didn't I tell him three times on the first night? The problem is not in him not hearing me, but in my own reluctance to communicate.

* * *

The weekly Shakti dancing class is having quite an impact on me. I see the same faces and, feeling more trusting of them, I realise I was in competition with women before. Isabella holds a consistently powerful space and is making me see how I'm not as empowered as I thought I was. I've been proving myself worthy with an impressive career and being really dynamic in order to feel accepted. All of the feminine qualities in me have been denigrated: softness, vulnerability, receptivity, emotionality. I'm not an empowered woman: I've been masculinised.

Isabella talks about our cyclical nature, and about being connected to the moon. Energy naturally moves outwards and inwards throughout the lunar phases. Our conditioning favours the outwards: giving and loving and caring, so we tend to neglect returning inwards. Each week we dance the different phases of the moon, each one a different archetype: warrior, mother, shaman, lover. I chart my cycle and notice how much I struggle with the shaman or 'shamana' as Isabella calls it in her Spanish accent, feminising the word. This is the premenstrual time when our energy is contracting as we cross the threshold into the dreamtime, to meet our unconscious. It's like a small death and has huge power and potential if we allow ourselves to descend.

184   MY BEAUTIFUL PSYCHOSIS

The shaman sees the truth in things and doesn't have time for nice-ties or social conventions. She's wild and connected, but our menstrual cycle has been seen as a curse. The intolerance and irritation, medi-calised as PMT, is actually a useful force to cull everything that's wrong in our lives. I notice how much I struggle at this time to be the dynamic go-getter personality I've invented for myself. It makes sense now why I would end up crying in a pub car park when I can't find my way to a business meeting in a place I haven't been to before. I shouldn't be bothering with such outward concerns when I'm dropping beneath the river beneath the river, as Clarissa Pinkola Estés calls it. It dawns on me that every single episode has started at this time of the month. Perhaps when I disappear into those strange states, I'm just going down to the unconscious.

The more I get in touch with my body in the dance, the less I feel like having sex with Ciaran. We have tried other ways. We worked through a Tantra book for a while but Ciaran thought it was boring. He refuses to listen to a talk about how to make love in a whole new way. *Making Love* explains how women have not been honoured enough and this is caus-ing relationships to break down and society to fragment. Sex should be a sacred act that connects two people intimately. It means being hon-est with each other about what's happening in the moment. The talk encourages couples to communicate with each other more so you both know what's going on and you're not in some fantasy in your head. Ciaran is always disappearing off into his. The lovemaking style takes the focus off chasing the orgasm and encourages presence and stillness, letting each moment lead authentically on to the next. It makes a lot of sense to me and I really want to give it a try, but Ciaran is adamant. He says that Barry Long, the speaker, is a sex addict and doesn't trust him.

* * *

Just reading *Practicing the Power of Now* is making me feel good. I admire Ekhart Tolle. The part I liked most in his first book, *The Power of Now*, was the introduction, where he mentions living on a park bench for a couple of years. He had been suicidal and thought he couldn't live with himself any longer. Then he had an epiphany: if he couldn't live with himself, then there was a Self and another self that he couldn't live with. Then he heard a voice in his head say, 'Resist nothing.' He awakened to the deepest sense of peace and presence that rendered him unable to function in the normal world, hence the park bench. Years later, he took the teachings from the experience and wrote them as a guide for others.

The Power of Now sold millions of copies because most people are living anywhere but now, including myself. I live in the future, worrying about what might happen, or I spend a lot of time imagining when things are better, fantasising. It's a form of self-medication. I also focus too much on what has happened and feel bad about it. My mind is so seductive and takes me off on an adventure that I follow. It just wants to fix everything with its problem/solution-oriented way of approaching life. Anything to avoid feeling how I feel in this moment right now. Even reading this book is a distraction because I'm using someone else's words to avoid my own thoughts altogether.

While I'm enjoying the teachings of Ekhart Tolle, Ciaran walks in, with a letter in his hand, looking shocked.

'We've got to move out. The landlord is coming back and wants to live here over the summer.' He passes me the letter. I feel totally calm, putting into practice *Practicing the Power of Now*. It's not happening now. It's a letter giving us two months. Right now we live in a large house that is expensive to run, which we have to sublet for office space and I'm happy to move on if we have to.

'Arsehole!' Ciaran attacks the person that is making him feel shit. Normally at this point I would soothe him and take care of his triggered trauma like a loving mother. But something stops me. I don't want to do that any more. Instead, I go into some blaming of my own: *Ciaran's ruining my practice. Why can't he just be more accepting of the situation? It's really no big deal. A minute ago I was at peace, but Ciaran has invaded my contentment with his petty drama.*

I close the book and put it back on the shelf. I could be happy in the present moment if it wasn't for other people.

CHAPTER TWENTY TWO

Workshop

Melissa has a way of describing events that makes me want to
go to them. She doesn't give any specifics, just says it will be
'amazing'. Melissa is a shiatsu client of mine but I can tell she
wants to be friends. I don't thrust the code of ethics at her but I do keep
a comfortable distance, not encouraging any connection outside our
sessions. Friendships are frowned on within a therapeutic relationship.
But this womb workshop she mentions sounds like something I want
to go to.

'It's with this *amazing* woman called Sophia.'

There are six of us in Sophia's home, a rented barn conversion in the
countryside, a few miles outside Totnes. Melissa's brought her husband
Tim with her. The only man. I'm not sure why he's come to a womb
workshop. I'm here because I feel disconnected from mine. And if that
is where my power is, then that's where I want to be. We do a guided
visualisation into the landscape of our womb, which takes us through
deserts and mountains and underwater caves until we reach a temple. I
see a Barbie-pink inflatable bouncy castle on the horizon. Not the lavish
structure I was hoping for. We are led into a great hall, up some steps
to an altar, which displays a golden egg. On the egg is a name. As I
approach I see the word 'Emma' written in my own hand. The 'E' is curly

and the letters are not joined up. It's how I wrote my name when I was ten years old. This, we are told, is our womb name. I'm relieved mine isn't a clichéd hippy one, the kind that people in Totnes have adopted, like Moonbeam or Eagle, but I'm a little concerned about its childlikeness. We're given the opportunity to share our experience with the others at the end, so I do.

'Oh, such innocence,' Sophia exclaims. Innocence? I hadn't thought of that.

Next we pair up with someone of a similar size for some Tibetan womb pulsing. My partner is a small, Asian-looking woman. Sophia demonstrates on her assistant. One person, the receiver, lies down on their back. The giver straddles them, sitting directly over their womb, and jolts up and down, like riding a horse. It looks simple enough, if a little embarrassing.

Sophia puts some music on to set the rhythm for us to follow. It's a rather intimate experience, which brings up a lot of sexual thoughts. It's not arousing as such, just the suggestion of the position and movement makes my head wander off into that territory. We manage to communicate enough to each other to establish the most effective angle and force and pound away for a good twenty minutes each. It's quite invigorating, and a lot of energy moves through my body. Suddenly, it feels like an atom bomb has exploded in my womb, sending out a boiling heat in its wake. But Melissa is struggling, and calls out to stop.

'It's bringing up old traumas.'

'It's just a story,' Sophia says. Maybe it is, but right now it's a story that's alive and running the show and you can't just brush that aside. I think it needs to be attended to with more compassion. Melissa's crying and gets up from the floor. Tim makes a kerfuffle, protecting his wife.

The woman next to me has a rather large and aggressive-looking woman on top of her. She's crying out in agony but is told to breathe through the pain. There's the pain of wrong position, and the pain of moving stuck energy, and they feel different. Maybe she doesn't trust herself enough to know which one this is, let alone guide her partner to a better angle.

The final exercise is another noisy one. We all lie on the floor side by side with our legs bent and feet beneath our knees, shoulder-width apart. Breathing in we call out 'ra' and then, outwards, 'hoom'. It's meant to access the vocal power in our wombs.

The woman next to me has quite a well to do accent and the way she says 'ra-hoom' tickles me. *Rah* like 'raj'. And *huuum* like 'humorous'. I think the *ra* is meant to be more of a 'roar' and *hoom* like 'boom'. I stifle a giggle, like a child at school that will get shouted at for disrupting the class. But posh lady's *rahhhh huuuuuum* next to me is getting louder. We sound so ridiculous: a bunch of middle-class white women all lined up in a row trying to vocalise the power of our wombs. *Raaaahhhhh huuuuuuum.*

I let out my laughter with full force. I don't care any more. It's just too funny. I'm roaring with my whole body and I might be mistaken, but it feels like it's actually coming from my womb. It's infectious and the others join in until everyone is laughing along with me and nobody knows why. Their howling is hollow and dry, dragged along by the force of my hilarity. The assistant looks like she's objecting to her giggles even as they leave her mouth. She gives Sophia a strange look, desperate, confused, and out of control with a questioning in her eyes. Still the room is a cacophony of guffaws giving me even more permission. The humour in the situation gets funnier the longer it goes on and I'm in no danger of running out of steam.

* * *

Since the womb workshop last weekend, I've not been sleeping so well. I can feel another episode coming on. It's the summer solstice full day of Shakti dancing this Saturday and I'm not sure if it's wise for me to go. I make it to the weekly drop-in class, now a regular fixture in my calendar, and talk to Isabella.

'It's better for you to be with other authentic women than on your own at home. You don't have to join in.' Isabella is quite convincing so I decide to go along, under the proviso that I can sit out if it feels too much for me.

The altar takes up most of the far wall and each woman has added a personal object, picture, or words of support on a piece of paper. The day is divided into the four archetypes: the mother, the warrior, the shaman, and the lover. The mother, who holds all, is the first round of the morning. Isabella puts on the now-familiar piece of music, *ReTURNING* by Jennifer Berezan, recorded in a six-thousand-year-old underground burial chamber in Malta. She guides us out of our heads and down into our bodies, encouraging us to let go. As usual, the tension in my face drops and my jaw rearranges itself. My groin does the same. I soften the soles of my feet and put my attention into each toe, unhooking any unconscious holding. With every tiny release, my shoulders also drop. I now feel more fleshy and pliable, flowing more easily through the space.

We pair up and sit opposite our partners on the floor, looking deep into each other's eyes. I feel blissful, and this beautiful woman who's sitting in front of me has a light in hers. She's at peace and enjoying my gaze as much as I'm enjoying hers. There's no need for words. There's no need for anything to mean anything. There's just this moment, here, now with this other being. A question arises in me, a bubble of curiosity popping to the surface of the still pond.

'What's your name?'

'Love,' she says and we both smile. I break out into gentle laughter and she joins me. Is that her real name? She might be answering from the place she's speaking from, the place we've both reached inside ourselves. But I wouldn't put it past someone in Totnes to actually be called Love.

Next, the warrior round, isn't where I'm at. Women are roaring but I'm still feeling the expansive unconditional love of the mother. I've raged at Ciaran in the past and been angry about a lot of things but right now I'm just not feeling it. Every sound the others are making is a stab in my belly. I decide to sit this one out and lean against the wall with my palms covering my solar plexus.

Isabella comes over and holds out her hand to me.

'Don't get stuck. No parking. Move it through.'

Am I stuck?

'I don't feel like dancing this one.'

'You're avoiding by sitting out. It's just a sabotaging strategy.'

Am I avoiding or just taking care of myself?

'I'm hungry,' I tell Isabella.

'You're angry,' she says back.

My stomach feels empty and it's well past lunchtime. If I'm angry, I'm not aware of it. But I guess Isabella knows best so I get up and rejoin the group.

Everyone has paired up again and this time we're encouraged to express our rage vocally to each other. The woman I'm with lets loose at me, flailing her arms and roaring like a lioness. Her expression drops to one of annoyance as she searches me for something to fight against but finds nothing. The longer she goes on without a response, the angrier she gets. I compose myself, looking directly into her eyes, open but somehow shielding myself from her rage. Whatever I'm doing is working because my belly is no longer jittery. She looks frustrated by my lack of anger and visibly gives up, roaring a final groan of irritation, like a child whose sibling won't play.

At half past two Isabella finally calls lunch. I switch my phone on to a series of worried messages from Ciaran. I don't feel like dealing with his anxieties right now. I think they're something for him to soothe in himself, so I switch it off again.

After lunch the lover round shows up my own difficulties with that particular archetype. I see Rachael, with her eyes closed, licking her lips erotically, her hips swaying and arms waving like an Indian goddess. For a second, she looks like a porn star, inviting sexual objectification and it makes me feel uncomfortable. I want to protect her and tell her to stop. But unlike porn stars, she's not faking it and deep down I really want to find that erotic lover in myself.

When the dance is over and the assistants are packing away, I sit in silence, not ready to face the approaching episode on my own. Isabella puts on some music to accompany the clear-up. The singer sounds like Rachael. The track seems to play over and over but I don't catch any of the lyrics.

Is it Rachael or am I hearing things?

Ciaran's away for the weekend so I get home to an empty house. He keeps texting to find out how I am and it feels overwhelming. I don't really know how to respond because I can't give him any reassurances so I don't respond at all. Instead I hunker down in my bedroom and get ready for the ride.

I contemplate calling Tanja to ask her to come over and midwife whatever is about to be birthed. I met Tanja the day Ciaran and I went to register our intention to marry. She was standing on the street chatting to Joe, Ciaran's Transition friend who got me the Transition film job. We crossed the road and told them our exciting news. I saw the energy in her chest flutter up to her face when she spoke to Ciaran. It was sexual. There's something in him that brings out the coquette in some women. Ciaran was once told that if he ever walked into a room and a saw a woman he was really sexually attracted to, he should get the hell out. It's how sex addicts find each other. I decided to make friends with Tanja. It was a conscious and calculated manoeuvre. What do they say about keeping your friends close but your enemies closer? Maybe calling her is not such a good idea. I probably need someone who's been through a spiritual emergency themselves and I don't know anyone around here who fits that bill.

A burning sensation takes centre stage in my solar plexus, like an incinerator blasting through that chakra. I've heard of something called a Kundalini awakening, when a serpent of energy, which lies dormant at the base of the spine, rises upwards and out of the head. It clears any blockages in its wake and many spiritual people do Kundalini yoga in the hope of activating it. I think that's what is happening. I probably have a block in my third chakra, just above the navel, which is hopefully being cleared. This third chakra is associated with the ego: the source of personal power, self-belief, and self-worth. It doesn't take much for it to become blocked. It may be the result of poor feedback, lack of affection, criticism, rejection, and being ignored or unappreciated. I hold my palm over the area to settle it a little, but it lasts most of the day. With it come unpleasant feelings of guilt and worry, accompanied by thoughts along those same lines. I remember when we worked on this chakra in shiatsu. One of the other students reported excruciating feelings of shame that lasted all evening. I ride them out, without acting on them, until eventually they subside.

I hear Rachael arriving, the gate squeaking, and her footsteps coming up the stairs.

'Hi Emma. Ciaran asked me to come and see how you are.' She sits herself down next to me crossing one leg over the other.

'You've crossed your legs.'

'Yeah.'

'Isabella says not to.' I haven't crossed my legs since I started Shakti dancing six months ago. It blocks the flow of energy.

'Oh well. I don't always do what Isabella says.'

I'm not sure what Rachael will make of me and I wonder what she'll report back to Ciaran. I'm not my usual social self. I don't invent a conversation to fill the gulf like I normally would. I don't have anything to say and I don't feel my usual awkwardness about that so we sit in silence.

We move outside into the garden. My belly is still on fire and blood flushes through my face bringing that emotion again that I don't recognise. I want to disappear down the black space under the shed so

I lie back and roll across the grass towards it. Rachael follows, tumbling over and over behind me. There's no way my body will make it in the narrow gap between the ground and the shed so I stop. Rachael stops too. It's a bit odd what she's doing but I prefer her copying me than restraining me.

By the time Ciaran gets home I keep slipping in and out of that other realm. A headless horseman, carrying his decapitated head under his arm, gallops towards me in the space about six feet in front of me. Though moving at quite a speed he doesn't actually get any closer. He looks like that light projection of Princess Leah in *Star Wars*. He's not physically solid and if I did reach out to touch him my hand would slip right through.

There's an oblong glass-topped coffee table along the wall of the living room. I slide under the surface and lie down on the wooden base. Like Snow White in her glass coffin waiting for her kiss, I close my eyes and lay my hands on my belly. Ciaran comes in and seeing me in the coffee table, ratchets up his concern to a whole new level.

The psychiatrist is now on his way. My fairytale has turned into a nightmare.

I don't know how to talk to the doctor when he arrives. He sits next to me on the bench outside, on the terrace. I can't function any more in consensus reality. An ambulance arrives and I'm put in a wheelchair and wheeled into the back. It is like riding in a spaceship very slowly, winding through the country lanes and out to Torbay Hospital.

'Doors opening. Doors closing.' The voice in the lift reminds me of an old school teacher, annunciating the letter 'o' like a 1950s BBC presenter. The hospital elevator takes us down. I'm now catatonic.

CHAPTER TWENTY THREE

Underworld

I find myself in a room on the female wing of Oak Ward, one of the two psychiatric units at Torbay Hospital. My bedroom door is propped open so a member of staff can sit in the doorway and watch me. Every few hours or so the shift changes and a different person is sitting there. The guardians of the underworld.

They flick through trashy gossip magazines and raise their eyes over the rim every now and again with a look that asks me if I'm ready to join them yet. *Grazia* has a place for me if I want it. The media monster is waiting for me, tempting me with the front cover, the ultimate contract. If I sign myself over, my every action will be in service of this empire, in exchange for eternal beauty in pictures. I don't even consider it.

Night-time brings a whole new scenario. In the corridor, just outside my now closed door, a game of craps is being played. I can hear each roll of the dice followed by a chalking up of the points.

Scratch scratch.

I know who it is. It's the fucking devil again, placing his bets as he plays for my soul.

The whole world is in on it. It's a global game being played out through scratch cards: men from every culture, addicted to the thrill of a chance of winning me, for sex. They buy their cards, sometimes over the phone, frantically rub off the golden coating, slathering like they're wanking off.

Scratch scratch.

Their tongues twist in their mouths and eyes bulge from their sockets, desperate to claim me to fulfil their sordid sexual fantasies and insatiable appetites.

Scratch scratch.

The morning light brings relief that I've survived the clutches of the dark side. Somewhere beyond the hospital, in the ether, on Cloud FM there's a party. Sophia and her assistant and a whole host of spiritual beings are celebrating me. Like a personal Live Aid, they've invited Robbie Williams and all the other mega pop stars. There's a stage and a massive crowd of people. I want to go! I want more than anything to see the audience cheering me on.

But I'm stuck here.

Two nurses busy themselves with my sheets, patting and tucking them in. Though silent, they have a connection between them that excludes me. They're just doing their job and I'm merely part of the furniture.

Suddenly I'm lying at the side of a muddy track. We're in a time before the roads have been paved, before cars were invented. Judging by my outfit I'm a man. I'm wearing a thick brown woollen cloak to keep me warm while travelling. My horse and carriage, if I was in one, is now nowhere to be seen. We've been stopped and somehow I've been thrown out and onto the ground. These two nurses, now in rough dark clothes are searching my pockets. They're robbing me in broad daylight.

Meanwhile, back in 2010, when they've finished rearranging my bedding, robbing me of my liberty and humanity, they leave my room, having not said a word.

I venture out into the corridor and onto the ward. There's a large open area by the main entrance. It's sunken with built-in, curved, cushioned seats and a couple of bookcases. Off that there are two rooms: a living room with the TV blaring out that no one is watching, and an art room. The art room door is open, so I go in. It's like a primary school classroom with multicoloured paper, all kinds of paints, glitter, and boxes full of stuff. I take some plain white paper and coloured pencils and sit on one of the chairs around the central table.

I don't normally draw or paint. I never feel inspired that way. Once, after I first took up qigong, a burst of creativity hit me and I explored painting the five elements I was learning in shiatsu: water, wood, fire, earth, and metal, abstract impressions of how the energy might look or feel. I was surprised with what I came up with. It was vibrant, dynamic, and alive.

I sit staring at the blank piece of paper in front of me. I reach for a green pencil and begin outlining the shape of the large canvas tent Ciaran and I bought with our wedding money. I don't remember exactly what it looks like so I use a little artistic licence. I picture it at the campsite on the Isle of Skye.

I spent two days in that tent on my own, while Ciaran went up the Cuillins. He took off with his backpack and some food, wanting wilderness and solitude: the wild man within. I didn't question being left behind, though I did resent it and wondered why he needed to make himself so separate. I felt bereft at first but I reconnected to myself listening to an online Awakening Women's Summit on my MP3 player, climbing my own internal mountain. Something shifted in me in those two days. The loneliness I felt in my relationship turned to a companionship with myself.

I concentrate intensely on the picture that's emerging, enjoying the repetitive movement of the pencils as I'm shading in. I complete one and begin another, this time in pastels. When I finish that one I start another one with watercolours. I like the focus and simple, repetitive action.

Another patient walks into the room and introduces herself. Gill doesn't seem that crazy. In fact she doesn't seem mad at all to me. She tells me she's here just for some time out, to avoid a crisis, as things were getting difficult at home. She picks out some shapes from a box labelled 'Make Your Own Stained Glass' and makes a start on a dolphin.

'When were you born?' she asks in a curious tone.

'October 17th, 1969.'

She writes it down as numbers and then adds them up $1+7+1+0+1+9+6+9 = 3+4 = 7$.

'Seven. *Yahweh.*'

'What do you mean?'

'You're the Second Coming of Christ.'

I'd never say this out loud, and certainly not on a psychiatric ward. It sounds like the most stereotypical thing a crazy person would claim to be.

'That's why I came in here: to meet you. It all makes sense now.'

I don't want to encourage her because I think we're all going to have to get there eventually: awaken to the Christ Consciousness that's in each and every one of us. I think we're all so much more than we imagine. Inside each of us is a Light. Babies are born with it. You can see it in their eyes. But gradually we forget. We're conditioned out of it.

'I can go home now.'

And with that she gives me the stained glass dolphin she's been working on, gathers up the rest of her decorations, and walks out of the art room.

Later I see one of the staff removing a star she's put on my bedroom door.

'We don't have favourites here so don't go putting anything on anybody else's doors, OK, Gill?'

After that, I don't see her again. She must have checked herself out.

I want to talk to someone about this Jesus thing. I want someone with authority to validate me, so I ask to see the chaplain. When she arrives, I suddenly get scared and have second thoughts. *What if she just thinks I'm insane, and blaspheming?*

'Are you Laura?' the chaplain asks as she approaches me. I shake my head and keep quiet about her having got my name wrong. I let her walk away looking confused. As I make my way back to my room, one of the other women on my ward walks out of her room and mouths something to me.

'*I see you.*'

She must have seen the movie *Avatar*. It's how the blue tribe greet each other, and means I see who you really are. I don't respond. I don't want to encourage people to project their power onto me. I'm nobody's saviour, and neither was Jesus. He was just modelling who we could all be. If Christ did return today, he'd probably be sectioned. I'm not going to let on that I have felt the Christ Consciousness until everybody else realises they have to awaken to it, too. Otherwise it's just asking for trouble. After all, thinking you're Jesus is a classic symptom of psychosis.

There's an older gentleman wandering around in a kilt. I don't think it at all odd but my parents find it weird.

'I'm Robert. Robert Hind.'

'Sorry? I didn't catch your surname.' His accent is so posh, the way he speaks through his nose makes it sound like Hound.

'Hind. H-I-N-D. *Hind.*'

'Hi Robert. I'm Emma.'

'Emma. Have you seen my brother around?'

'No, sorry, I haven't.'

'You look like my first wife.'

'Oh.'

'Yes, we married in 1964 and separated in 1982. Then I met my second wife. She was born in 1955 and we separated in 1995.' As he talks, he steps from one foot to the other in a beat that I'm feeling in my own body. I don't know if it's his medication or the rhythm of the universe.

'Then my third wife was born in 1967 and we married in 1998. We separated in 2004.' Robert's stepping from side to side gradually backs me into the corner of the courtyard.

'I notice your wives get younger,' I say, inching away from the wall, round the other side of him so we change places.

'Have you met my brother? He's wearing a kilt.'

It suddenly dawns on me that *he* is his brother. He probably has multiple personality disorder.

'No, Robert. I haven't met your brother.'

'Look this is awfully embarrassing as I seem to have come to the hospital without my slippers. And they won't let me out you see. If I gave you some money perhaps you could purchase some from the shop for me.'

'I don't think I'm allowed out either, Robert, but my parents are coming later today and I'll hopefully go out with them. What's your budget?'

'Here take this.' He hands me a five pound note. 'Nothing too fancy. I'm having to walk around in my socks, which won't do at all.'

When my parents arrive, we go for a walk on a path that goes all the way around the perimeter of the hospital grounds. We stop at a picnic table where Mum and Dad take some sandwiches out of their rucksack. As they're eating, I walk over to a large pine tree and stand beneath.

That horrible weird, dark feeling takes hold of me and pulls me into myself. I can't move. I'm stuck, shrinking and shrinking into a black pit. Dad comes over and reaches his hand under the branches. I take hold of it and let him slowly pull me out. Then the feeling is gone.

There aren't any slippers in the shop, just crisps and newspapers and sweets and stuff.

'Sorry, Robert. I could only go to the shop near the hospital reception and they didn't have any slippers.' I hand him back his money.

'Not to worry.' He pauses before asking, 'What do you do?'

'I'm a filmmaker.'

'I'm making a film about my recovery. It's called Robert's Recovery. I've got some photos I'll show you.'

'That sounds great,' I lie.

'I'm setting up an organisation and I think you would make a good treasurer. I have lots of contacts. Here, take this to start us off. Keep it safe.' He hands me back the fiver, which I reluctantly put in my pocket. I don't want to force him out of his fantasy world. I'll find a way to get his money back to him before I leave.

Phil Hudson is quite a character. He's loud and likes to draw attention to himself. The staff plays up to him, laughing at his jokes. He keeps changing his hairstyle and today he's gone for a footballer's short Mohican. It must be something to do with the World Cup. We're standing in the main hallway talking. Well, he's talking and I'm listening. There's a piece of fluff sticking out of his nose and it flutters every time he breathes out. I reach up and gently remove it.

'That was really intimate,' he declares turning my gesture into more than it was.

'Was it?'

'Yes. The way you just did that. It was so intimate. You like me! You like me don't you? *Ha!*'

'What makes you think I didn't like you?' I say, hopefully removing the idea of any sexual interest but keeping the like as a 'friend's kind of liking'.

Joan—a recent admission—walks up the ramp towards the front door and tries to open it, but it's locked. Both Phil and I turn to watch.

'Let me out,' she calls, probably hoping a member of staff in the office will hear and come over with the key. When nobody responds she calls out again.

'Let me out. I want to see my kids. *LET ME OUT!*'

'She only arrived yesterday. She's not allowed out I expect,' Phil says, turning back to look at me. Joan's getting quite worked up.

'LET ME OUT. I NEED TO SEE MY CHILDREN. THEY'LL BE WONDERING WHERE I AM.' Joan pulls repeatedly on the door until she attracts a member of staff.

'I'm sorry but we can't let you out.' The nurse is calm but I can tell he's covering up his fear.

'BUT I NEED TO SEE MY KIDS. I ONLY CAME IN AFTER A MAD NIGHT OUT. I'M OK NOW. YOU'VE GOT TO LET ME OUT TO SEE THEM.'

'I'm sorry but I can't do that. I can't let you out. You're being assessed by the doctors. You're not allowed out until they give us the all clear. Calm down. I can't open the door for you. Come away. Go back to your room. Can I get some help over here?'

A second member of staff comes over. There's no way she's going to be let out but she keeps on in desperation.

'*Please*, you've got to let me out to see my children.'

'You just watch, they're going to drag her off and forcibly medicate her. They did that with me once but I concentrated hard and pushed all the *chi* down into the ground so I weighed a tonne and it took four men to carry me. That's what they're going to do. They'll take her down the corridor and into her room and hold her down on the bed and inject her with Largactil and then she'll go quiet because it's like an elephant tranquilliser and she'll be asleep for hours and when she wakes up she'll feel like shit. They just want to control us, make us passive and easier to manage.'

Phil is talking non-stop, in my face, barely pausing for breath. Meanwhile in the background the staff must be getting rougher because I can hear Joan sounding screechy now as well as loud.

'Get off me. Get your hands off me. Ow. That hurts. GET OFF ME.'

Both conversations are happening at once. I'm looking at Phil and I can't see Joan behind me but I stretch out my attention wide so I can hear them equally: Phil in my face talking loudly and Joan screaming in the background.

'Told you—they're taking her to her room and there won't be a peep out of her until tomorrow. She'll go quiet once they've medicated her. It's so fucked up.'

'YOU'VE GOT TO LET ME OUT OF HERE. I NEED TO SEE MY CHILDREN. OPEN THE FUCKIN' DOOR. I'M PERFECTLY OK. IT WAS JUST A MAD NIGHT. GET OFF ME.'

Mayhem in stereo. The kerfuffle moves along the corridor with Joan complaining all the way. The two members of staff don't speak, relying instead on physical force.

Then it all goes quiet.

'You're so calm. How come you're so calm?' Phil asks me. 'You're a good influence on me.'

* * *

Robert Hind is chewing my ear off and pacing from side to side with his strange poetic rhythm. I have no interest in what he's saying. He, like Phil, is unable to be quiet and calm.

'Robert. I bet you five pounds you can't keep quiet for five minutes.'

'OK. I bet you I can.'

'Go ahead, then.' Robert checks his watch and shows me the time. He makes a gesture to zip up his lips. I'm left watching the twitching dance of his feet. I figure out the beat. Dum, dumdedum, dum, da da dum. It's a four bar beat whose waves I feel through my body.

I discovered, while studying shiatsu, that I'm an empath. This means I feel what other people are feeling. Sometimes my throat closes up when I touch on a client's grief. As soon as they access it in themselves, the feeling inside me disappears. It's a useful tool as a therapist but can be confusing in social situations.

Robert is quiet while sliding from side to side in his odd way. The rhythm is probably the effects of his medication, I decide, before looking at the time.

'Your five minutes are up Robert. Well done!'

And I give him back his five pound note.

CHAPTER TWENTY FOUR

Confession

I want to walk home across country rather than go in the car. Dad insists that we should drive part of the way through the built-up area until we get to Marldon and then walk the green lanes to Berry Pomeroy. But newly built houses have hidden the route to the footpath. We search the village and can't find a way through, though there's a path clearly marked on the map. It's a mystery we don't solve and I resign myself to the inevitable car ride, pissed off that nobody else seems to care about keeping our precious footpaths open.

Once home I potter around preparing to move house. There's a lot of packing up to do and sorting through what we'll need to store. We're moving back into the annexe across the road, where we moved from in the first place. We've accumulated a lot of furniture, which we don't want to get rid of, so it all has to go into storage.

When I see Rachael again, I thank her for taking care of me while Ciaran was away.

'I've been wondering about something. At the end of the summer solstice Shakti dance, I heard a track that I thought was you. Was that you singing, because I didn't recognise the song?'

'Yes. It was something Isabella commissioned me to record for her friend's birthday. It's called *Emotional Creature*. It's a poem by

Eve Ensler. I can give you a copy of it if you like.' She does, and I play it immediately.

It's a celebration of woman's ability to feel emotions. Somewhere along the way I have learnt to stuff my feelings down and be in my head. Through the socialisation process when growing up, through my family's unconscious and unspoken agreement to brush things under the carpet and be happy, through an overemphasis on thinking in the education system, through a cultural pressure to be polite and an expectation that women should be 'nice', my feelings have never been valued. But here they are, being described as the very thing that makes me better. When I struggle with insomnia, my mind awash with thoughts invading my head, I've found that feeling my emotions does make me better. It takes me out of my head and back into my physical body, joining me back up, disconnected parts coming back together, making me feel whole again.

Studying shiatsu I learnt about the damage that blocked emotions can cause. I watched as Ken demonstrated on willing and eager students, how freeing them up resulted in the immediate cessation of their symptoms. He taught us how to access them in our bodies by bringing our attention to our bodily sensations, including and especially any physical pain. I witnessed the release of old traumas that had been causing aches and stiffness for years. A niggling tension in my back, when felt with focus and acceptance, was a rage so ferocious, the rising energy burst blood vessels in my eyes. Letting go of these stuck feelings, I came to believe, is the key to curing many symptoms such as back pain, headaches, digestive problems and even anxiety. I discovered that my anxiety was simply the quivering of my nervous system keeping a lid on my emotions. As soon as I've released the anger and grief beneath, the anxiety disappears. So emotions are not only to be celebrated in women but encouraged in everyone as an essential component to health.

If I ask why emotions are denigrated and seen as an inconvenience in women, the answer is political. It allows the continued decimation of this planet's delicate ecosystem, destroying natural habitats, depleting species, changing the atmosphere and thus climate, the continued stealing of lands from tribal people for access to resources and violent conflict and wars over these resources. It's a mighty inconvenient truth indeed. If we all felt the true depths of pain that this causes, we could not and would not continue to inflict it. The only way we can keep our global economy going is by denying and ignoring and avoiding this pain. Avoiding our feelings is the underlying cause of addiction and we're all addicted to something if we're honest enough with ourselves: coffee, sugar, alcohol, television, games, running, shopping, gambling, painkillers, painkillers all. It's what our consumer economy depends upon. You will feel better if you buy … (*fill in the blank*).

I play the track again and again, crying all the way through. By the third listen I'm singing along, celebrating myself and all that I've been through: all that I feel and it's all OK.

* * *

Our relationship is not going well. Ciaran wants us to see a psychotherapist, saying we're in crisis. I don't feel particularly in crisis. I feel empowered, autonomous, and able to stand my ground. I'm happy plodding along building my new filming business and deepening my friendships with the other Shakti dancers. I'm not taking care of him like I used to, and I think he's struggling with that.

Isabella offers us some sessions as she and her partner work with couples. I suggest it to Ciaran but he has a reaction. He knows her partner and he has judgements about him. We talk about going to see a sexual therapist but we can't find one that comes highly recommended. In any case, he seems to be set on a particular psychotherapist who's got a good reputation. I don't feel like I need therapy but I go along for a trial session with Ciaran to make sure I'm not just being stubborn. Afterwards I still don't feel the need to go as a couple but suggest he goes on his own if he thinks it will help. Whatever helps him will surely be of benefit to the relationship. When he comes back from his sessions I always ask how they went and what they explored.

By September we're still no closer, and I don't know what to do. I'm at a loss as to how to move forward. Ciaran has found a couples' counsellor that everyone around here seems to go to. I agree to go as a way of figuring out whether we should stay together or not. We're not talking about splitting up, but just going with this question in mind as a starting point.

Hannah, our counsellor, suggests we look at our family backgrounds. She has a big flipchart and allocates us a page and a session each. We begin with Ciaran's family, going through all his significant members back to his grandparents. Hannah draws them out like a family tree and links each person to Ciaran with the words he uses to describe their relationship. Ciaran takes much longer than the allotted single session to make his way through the complexity that is his ancestry.

When it's my turn, I feel a little ordinary by comparison. Ciaran appears bored having to sit through my turn even though I take up half the time he did. Hannah is confused looking at the diagrams side by side and can't see anything obvious that stands out to her. I think perhaps the whole exercise is a waste of time and money. It's not really helping us decide about our relationship.

In the next session I remember that Mum had a brother that I didn't include in my family tree. The story I've heard about him is that he went off to the army and when he returned he was a different man. He had become an alcoholic and neglected his children. He set fire to his house and ended up in prison, while the kids were taken into care. Mum's parents kept giving him chances but he repeatedly stole from them until eventually they distanced themselves from him. He died when I was a teenager. My mother hadn't seen him for years, and I never met him.

Hannah's face looks like a penny has dropped.

'That's the connection I was looking for. It makes sense now. Your family trees didn't match up before but that's the missing piece.'

Apparently ancestral wounds get carried down the line for generations, replaying themselves out until they're recognised and healed. Perhaps I've attracted Ciaran in order to heal the wounds of my mother's family. It's a revelation I'm not sure what to do with. Mum has always enjoyed the story of Ciaran's redemption. Maybe it's because her brother never redeemed himself. I hadn't made the link before, that he was filling the gap left by this banished uncle. The universe abhors a vacuum. If I've married Ciaran because of this familial split then I'm not so much repeating the pattern of my family as trying to help us to become more whole. But where does that leave Ciaran and me?

'Emma, you talk about wanting a different kind of sex life. What is it that you want?' Hannah asks me.

'I want sex to be sensuous and intimate. For it to feel sacred, spiritual even. I want to tune into energy and follow that, letting it lead the way. I want it to be more connected.'

'I'm curious, Ciaran. How much of that did you hear as a criticism?'

'Pretty much all of it.' Hannah is astute. I had no idea that telling Ciaran what I wanted led to him feeling criticised.

* * *

Lustleigh Cleave isn't a part of Dartmoor I know well. I usually like to use a guidebook and do a circular route. But Ciaran prefers to be more adventurous and walk wherever he likes. There's a right to roam on the moor so you don't have to stick to the paths but this means difficult terrain. I can't stand having to look down at my feet all the time, lifting my legs higher than usual to step over the ground cover. It's tiring and irritating.

We stop for a flask of peppermint tea, sinking into the cushion of heather.

'There's something I have to tell you.' Ciaran pauses but I say nothing, waiting for the bad news.

'In telling you I might lose everything but it might lead me to getting everything I ever wanted.' Another pause as he gathers himself. 'I've been unfaithful.'

'What?' A cold fog coagulates in my head, freezing any emotion.

'When we were in Bristol for that wedding. I went round to see Laura. I knew it was a mistake. I knew what was going to happen. I felt awful afterwards. We didn't have penetrative sex.' Laura is a friend of his who came to our wedding. She spoke about how difficult her marriage was at my hen do.

I still don't say anything. I can't. I'm in shock.

'My psychotherapist encouraged me to tell you because of our counselling sessions. She said it's not right to keep something from you given that we're sharing a truthful space.' He pauses again but still I say nothing.

I'm picturing us dancing at my friend's wedding, kicking our legs out forwards and backwards in unison and smiling at each other. I felt really happy in that moment, sharing some fun with Ciaran again. And all along he was feeling terrible for what he'd just done. His smiling face was a lie. I make a quick calculation in my head. It was three weeks ago. We'd had one session with Hannah by then. It must be some sort of reaction to the couples counselling. I know that whenever we take a step to deepen our relationship in some way, one of us usually has a wobble, a form of sabotage driven by unconscious fears of intimacy.

'I'm also telling you because you knew anyway. You weren't conscious of it but I could see it was making you a little crazy so I thought I'd better tell you.'

'I need to go.' I pack up the rucksack and sling it on my back. I head back to the car, abandoning the walk.

Fury hits me when I get back to the house.

'You didn't have penetrative sex? You think saying that lessens the blow? All it does is give me an image of her sucking you off. So what did you do together? Did she give you a blow job?'

'I'm not going to go into the details of it.'

'No but you're quite happy to tell me what you didn't do as if it gets you off the hook. And with Laura! She sat in my sacred circle of women at my hen do. She's a shiatsu practitioner too.'

'She's a liability.'

'*You're* the fucking liability, Ciaran. I need you to go. You'll have to find somewhere else to live until I've figured this out.'

Ciaran doesn't argue. He makes some calls and finds a bell tent on someone's land he can stay in. We only have one car so I drive him there, leaving him looking shocked and forlorn in a white, empty space with only a small bag of essentials. I don't know how long it will be for. I need to be away from the ridiculous things he says, which aren't helping. I also want him to experience having left the relationship because that is effectively what he's done.

After three weeks with Ciaran in the doghouse, my anger turns to pity and I invite him to come back home. I still haven't decided about whether I want to stay with him or not. I always imagined that if he was unfaithful we would work it out. I understand Ciaran and his addictions and I know that his infidelities are not what he really wants. But now that it's happened I don't feel so sure I want to stay with him. I'm not really happy in this relationship.

* * *

Shilpa's someone I met through Ciaran. She was married to an addict friend of his, who died of an accidental overdose. I made a short film for her a while ago, but our friendship hasn't really blossomed until now. Her husband was also a sex addict. She lends me a book about love addiction. It claims that behind every sex addict is a love addict. It obviously struck a chord with her because otherwise why would she think it might be useful to me? The unspoken implication is that I must be a love addict too.

The book describes many scenarios of women who keep taking the sex addict back even though he clearly cannot remain faithful. The love addict sounds like rather a pathetic creature willing to put up with a lifetime of shit. That, I'm clear, is not me. There's no way I'm going to count myself among their number.

At our next session with Hannah I declare emphatically that I know I can't handle another infidelity in the future. When I say it, I can feel how true it is. It's not a threat, just a knowing of my limits.

'And I can't handle another episode.' Ciaran swallows hard. He's not trying to get one over on me. He means it, too. We're actually both in the same boat.

* * *

Woods is not a café I usually hang out in. In fact I've never been before. It was Rebecca's suggestion and I'm not really bothered where we meet. Seeing my friends has become even more important as I navigate, what seems like now, a situation I should have seen coming. They are all really supportive and no one judges Ciaran, though he projects that onto them. He worries that everyone hates him now and his reputation is in tatters. He shows no concern for how I might be feeling in all of this.

As we sit facing each other, sipping herbal tea, something stirs at the bottom of my belly.

'I think I have to leave Ciaran,' I say a little unsure, trying on the words for size. As I say them, a powerful force rises up from my womb, the knowing that I've been waiting for. I'm not sure if it's riding on the wake of the words or the words are pushed up by its power. It's not a head kind of knowing, nor even a heart one, because I start to cry as soon as I hear myself utter it. My heart could never make this kind of decision. Rebecca watches me in silence, witnessing this profound moment of truth. I don't cry for long. I'm going to need all the strength I can find.

I don't know how I'm going to tell Ciaran. I feel guilty, giving up on our marriage, giving up on him. For some reassurance I go to see a psychic medium. Karen only knows my first name, which I told her on the phone as I made the booking. I haven't mentioned anything else about my life. I'm curious to know how much she'll pick up on without my prompting. She's an attractive young woman with lots of jangly bracelets and a short skirt. Her dark hair is wavy and layered, rock chic with tattoos poking out from under her clothes. Her voice is hoarse from too much smoking.

'I use a guide who's quite blunt. He just tells it like it is so my apologies in advance for that. It's not me being rude. It's just how he communicates.'

She hands me a pack of tarot cards and asks me to shuffle them.

'Go to India! He's telling me you should go to India.'

I've been invited to go to India twice recently by two different friends, Shilpa and Rachael, but I've declined. I was born in India and have been back once with a school trip when I was eighteen. I do want to go but with all that's been happening with Ciaran I haven't felt it was the right time. I don't want to go as a way of running away.

Karen turns over the death card.

'Now people get the wrong idea about this card. It doesn't mean you're going to die. You're going through a major transformation, a dying of your old self. You need to leave your husband.'

'Right.'

'But you're embarrassed about it. Why are you embarrassed about it?'

'I've only been married two years.'

'He's not been faithful to you. You'll meet someone else.'

'Will he find somebody new?'

She turns over another card.

'Yes.'

I feel relieved. She gives me a description of Ciaran that is incredibly accurate and reiterates that I should go to India.

'You have a South American woman guiding you at the moment, M... M... I can't pronounce it so I'll just call her Maria. She's describing a past life you had together and how beautiful her funeral was.' Karen goes into some details about the occasion but I've lost interest. I don't know this Maria woman and wonder why she's hogging my session with memories of her passing.

'She's here to help you open your heart. And then someone called Steve will take over.'

I don't have a conscious connection with any spirit guides so this information could be entirely made up. She's picked up and confirmed my need to leave Ciaran and that's what I came for. But I still don't know how I'm going to tell him.

'What did she say about us?' Ciaran asks me when I get home.

'I'm not telling you. Why don't you go and see her yourself?' Maybe if he has a session with Karen he'll hear it from her. Ciaran books himself in but when he returns he's not as impressed as I was.

'She's full of shit.'

'Well she got you off to a tee. What did she say about us?' It's my turn to be curious.

'She told me I had to stick at my marriage. What the fuck does she know?'

So that's why he didn't like her. He seems annoyed by the idea of having to work at our marriage. I'm confused and disappointed. I thought she told the future. I was hoping she would tell him that his wife was going to leave him. This means I'm going to have to tell him myself. I guess we both got guidance according to what's best for each of us. It's probably in Ciaran's highest interests to stick at it but the most growth for me is in leaving.

I don't want Ciaran to get angry when I tell him. The trick is to make it seem like it's his idea too. So one Sunday morning, as we're having a lie-in, I glance over at the photo on our bedside table. We're lying curled up together in a pink nylon tent that's reflecting off our skin. We look rose-tinted.

'I don't remember feeling like that. Do you?' I nod my head towards the picture.

'No.'

'It's like it's somebody else.' I stare into the image of two happy people in love.

'Maybe we should separate.'

Ciaran couldn't agree fast enough. If he suggested a separation to me I would have been really upset. It's as if he's been waiting for an excuse to give up on us.

I book a flight to India departing on April 12. Then I realise that it's the anniversary of the day that Ciaran and I first met. Six years exactly. It gives us three months to get used to the idea of parting and for me to find somewhere else to live. These three months are quite blissful. Ciaran and I are very loving and tender with each other and there are no arguments. I no longer need anything from him and that's freed me up to just love him as he is. As my departure time approaches, I can't help wondering if we might actually be able to work it out.

'Are we doing the right thing?'

'Of course.' Ciaran doesn't seem to share my doubts.

The day before I fly out to Delhi, I still haven't found anywhere suitable to live. I've seen a notice pinned to a lamppost in town and arranged to go and look at the place. Everywhere in Totnes is quite expensive but this is a one-bed with an extra attic space, water and council tax included for only £495 a month. Ciaran comes with me for moral support.

A smiley man with glasses answers the door and welcomes us in. He leads us upstairs and shows us around. It's an ex-council house on an estate just out of town. The rooms are small and boxy but that will just make it cheaper to heat. I'll be able to sleep in the attic and then what was the bedroom can be my office. It's perfect.

'I'll take it.'

'Great. We knew you were the one when you called.'

'Can I give you a cheque for the deposit?'

'Sure.'

'I fly off to India for a month tomorrow so can you hold it for me until the 13th of May when I come back?'

'Absolutely. I'm a little confused, though. Will it be the two of you, or just you?'

'No, it's just me.'

The landlord looks at us both questioningly.

'We're separating.'

'Oh.'

He has a contract on the kitchen table ready for me to sign. I check the address. The postcode ends in exactly the same three letters as my parents' house I grew up in. I take it as a good sign, the spirit world helping me along.

Ciaran drives me to the train station and waits with me on the platform. Heading off for an adventure to Dharamsala, the home of the exiled Dalai Lama; exploring Rishikesh, the place that spiritually influenced The Beatles; and trekking to the source of the Ganges is softening the blow of our relationship ending.

My train pulls in and I step on board, closing the door behind me. I push down the window and hold my hand out of the carriage. Ciaran takes it in his and smiles at me with wet eyes. I love him so much. His boyish good looks, his soft nut-coloured hair, his big shining hazel eyes and tall frame. But most of all I love his smile. It lights up his face and changes his whole outlook.

I'm leaving with mixed emotions. I don't want to go but I feel I have to. Ciaran's infidelity was a symptom of the breakdown in our relationship rather than the cause. I can't blame it all on him and his sex addiction, though that looms large as a major factor. It's really just the catalyst. If I had to pick a moment when it all changed, the turning point, it was the moment I decided not to soothe him any more: when we got the letter from our landlord saying we had to move. I've helped him through many challenges and he's appreciated my skill at that. It's how he made me feel valued. But that's really a form of co-dependence. If one of you changes and stops doing that thing that keeps the relationship going then it can go one of two ways: either the other person changes as well, or the relationship breaks down. For us it's the latter.

My episodes are destabilising for Ciaran and they are happening every two years. They trigger the old wound inside him of being abandoned by his mother when he was only two years old. Soon after we first met, and before he'd experienced me in an episode, we had an important conversation about them. I made it very clear that I thought it was a spiritual crisis and I needed people not to pathologise my state of mind. I keep my experiences closeted from the mental health services because they interpret everything as a symptom. I need to be with someone who respects and shares my perspective and treats me accordingly. It's a deal breaker.

When the train moves off we're still holding hands, and Ciaran wipes the tears from his face with his free hand. He walks along the platform following alongside the train. I make a deliberate gesture of letting go, splaying my fingers out and humming the title music to *Six Feet Under*. There's a shot in the title sequence where two elderly hands suddenly part, representing another death. We've watched the entire six series of this American TV show together. There's a shiatsu practitioner in it who turns out to be a sex addict. It's *our* show. Ciaran laughs.

'Perfect timing,' he says and I laugh with him and then wave. When he's out of sight, I turn away and find my seat.

EPISODE SEVEN

CHAPTER TWENTY FIVE

Medium

Marjory Matthews is a very busy medium. I've had to wait two months for my appointment with her. Now that Ciaran and I are properly separated, I need some reassurance that I've done the right thing. I still love him and light up whenever I see him. We're sharing our car at the moment, which gives me an excuse to pop round when I have to drop it off. He's moved in with a friend just five minutes walk around the corner. I think I'm just weaning myself off him gradually but I wonder whether we could have made it work if I'd tried harder.

Marjory is a beautiful older woman with a friendly round face and a light in her eyes. She has a slight Midlands accent, though she lives in North Devon.

'I've got to say now that while you were outside, sitting on the bench, there was someone sitting beside you. Somebody who's died.'

'Which side?' I ask abruptly, partly to catch her out, partly curious about whether they're on my masculine (right) or feminine (left) side.

'I don't know. I just noticed they were sitting beside you. They're standing right beside you at the moment.' She's gesturing towards my right.

'Oh. OK. Do you know who it is?'

'I don't yet. They haven't told me who they are yet. Someone who didn't get a chance to say goodbye anyhow.'

'I don't actually know many people who've died.'

'This person is not a relative of yours. It's someone that ... all I can say is that there's a connection and you've known each other and you may have been friends. You may have even had a relationship. It's a male. I know he died suddenly. But hadn't seen you for quite some time.'

I can't think who it is so Marjory changes the subject. She tells me I've got big changes around me that will alter the course of my life. She mentions a contract being on its way and I think about the Transition Network, who have asked me to make another film. So much has happened in the world of Transition that they want to showcase since the first film was released. She also tells me that television is on the horizon for me.

'But you need to be the real *you*, Emma. Don't be the people pleaser. You've done that too much and people have treated you like a doormat. And you're too good for that. Don't do it again. You're a very spiritual lady. You are spiritually led. Everything you do is spiritually led. You're actually very gifted. Wonderful healing in your hands, by the way. Are you aware of that?'

'I'm a shiatsu practitioner.'

'Ah well, no wonder. Even in the creative side of your life you heal. You do things that create healing, don't you?'

'I try.'

'Don't ever stop doing this work. In one form or another. Because it's what you came into this life for. You came here to tell a story. And that's what your work will do, tell stories.'

It feels good to hear all this about my healing hands and my life purpose. I like the idea that I came here to tell a story. Marjory goes back to the subject of the spirit who is apparently with me.

'Um. This young man beside you has got the initial C. Like Craig. Or it might be his surname.'

'No. I don't know.'

'He said, 'She knows me! She knows me!''

'Sorry.' I cry out into the space where he's apparently standing. 'I know a lot of people.' Marjory and I both laugh.

'He's not really bothered. He came along because he knew you were coming today.'

'Just for a laugh.'

'Let's have a laugh at Emma's expense.' We giggle together and I warm to her. 'Whoever he is he's got a sense of humour, and he died suddenly.'

'OK.'

'I think he died in a motor accident,' Marjory adds.

'Oh, I know. I think I know. A long time ago,' I respond, remembering.

'Yeah. He said this is the first opportunity to be spoken to.' As Marjory says this, she says it in exactly the same way my first boyfriend, Ian Clapp, would have said it.

'If it's the guy I'm thinking of, I was only about fourteen at the time. What does he want, then?'

Marjory explains that his task in this part of his life is to help souls who feel lost. When he heard I needed help he wanted to be the one to do it because he knew me. Apparently I wasn't a complete lost soul but I was losing myself.

'He's like an angel without wings. Lovely man,' Marjory says.

'Can I check the name so I've got the right person?'

'Yeah.'

'I think it's Ian.'

'What was his surname?' Marjory asks.

'Clapp.'

'That's it! He was doing this to me first of all.' Marjory does an exaggerated clapping gesture with her hands. 'And I didn't take any notice. He said, "I can help you with whatever you need."'

'Ah. That's nice.'

'And he said, "It's our pleasure. My pleasure."'

I went out with Ian in the summer holidays on our first trip back from Hong Kong. He must have been about fifteen or sixteen, a year or two older than me. He had floppy blond hair and a soft, friendly face. I remember hanging around the village, leaning against a lamppost with his arm around me. We didn't say very much but that didn't matter. He drove me around on the back of his motorcycle while I clung on, trying not to clunk his helmet whenever he touched the brakes. He took me water-skiing for the first time and even treated me to a meal in a posh restaurant. We must have looked cute dining out together at our age. I never worried about him trying anything on with me like other guys. We wrote to each other for quite a while when I returned to Hong Kong in September. His letters apologised for his terrible English and explained how writing them was helping him. He wasn't motivated to improve his spelling and grammar before, but now he had a good reason to. One letter talked about a friend of his that was killed in a motorbike accident. The parents gave Ian a talking to about the dangers on the road so he got rid of his bike after that. He sent me a single of Stevie Wonder *I Just Called To Say I Love You* but he sent it overland so it took six weeks to arrive. He was the sweetest boyfriend I ever had.

'There's happiness here for you. And a sense of being settled in a relationship. A relationship that you'll feel secure in. But with somebody that isn't a liar. Have you had an on-off relationship with someone?'

'I've just separated from my husband.'

'Oh, that's what it is. I can see it being switched on and then off again. He isn't a bad person. Not at all. He's a good man in many ways. But the sense is that he's quite a busy man. And it feels as if he puts too much of himself into his work and very little of himself into a relationship. He thinks he puts lots into a relationship. But actually he doesn't. His mind is but his actions aren't. He still loves you. I think he's trying not to. But he still loves you. Ah, thank you. This young man you've got with you in spirit, Ian. He said, "This is what we've been supporting her through." I think your husband had eyes for someone else.'

Marjory describes the effect that this has had on me. How it made me feel insecure and damaged my self-esteem.

'He's a controller, this man. You were controlled by your husband because you allowed yourself to be, because you didn't see yourself as important as a person. You've got a long life ahead of you. It's time you stepped up to the plate and start living it instead of just existing it.'

'I've got health issues. Mental health issues.'

'I think if you start liking the woman you are those will go. You need to like her otherwise you can become paranoid. And you're not paranoid. But it's not a very long journey for you to go there.'

Marjory suddenly changes the subject and tells me that I was conceived a twin. This is news to me. Apparently we knew that both of us couldn't survive. Only one of us could come, otherwise neither of us would have made it. We would have got almost to the birth and then died. So we played a game to decide who would come.

'And you lost. You came.'

'I lost,' I blurt, laughing at the cosmic joke.

'You lost, yeah.' Marjory laughs too. 'But your sister would be your guardian angel. I hadn't seen her until this moment.'

'My mother's first pregnancy was twins. They both died.'

MEDIUM 221

'Well that was the two of you trying to come the first time. And you came back again. And that's why you've always felt that you're not good enough. It's why you feel guilty for all sorts of reasons. No reason at all sometimes. And it's why you're always lonely. You're missing your twin.'

Marjory's losing me a little with this twin thing. Everything else she's said has been spot on but I'm not really sure how this relates to my experiences of spiritual emergency or psychosis, or whatever.

'I don't think you have a mental health problem. I really don't. From what I can see it's a childhood embryo stage problem. It's before you came into this life. It's the womb time. You're not bipolar.'

'Well, that's one of the labels.'

'You're not bipolar. And you're not manic depressive. My feeling is that you can take control of this. I think stop letting anyone control you. You take control of this and say, "I know where this is coming from." I don't feel worried about you and your mental health. People like to put labels on us.'

'A lot of it feels like a really intense spiritual experience that I get scared of.'

'I think it is spiritual. They tried to put me away.' Marjory tells me a funny story about when her parents took her to see a psychiatrist. She was only little and didn't know what a psychiatrist was. During her appointment, she saw his little boy who had died so she told the doctor.

'He told my parents I had ESP and I went, "Is it catching?" So I totally understand. People thought I was crazy because I could see dead people. I was only nine or ten. You're not going crazy. Do you wonder whether it's a dream or reality?'

'Yeah. To the outside world I've become catatonic but what's happening to me is I've entered another realm of existence where it's kind of ... where there's a whole other level of everything going on and there's too much I don't understand.'

'You step out of this dimension. That's what happens to you there. When that happens again you need to start asking questions. Say, "OK, tell me what this is all about?" It's no good just being the viewer. I've got this thing where I go off into another place and I don't know whether I'm dreaming or whether I'm awake. And yet a large part of me knows I'm awake. And then I'll think, *is this real or is it a dream*? Does that make sense?'

'And also with mine, there's a whole ancestral backlog as well.'

'Oh, you're seeing past. So you have the ability to read past lives. That's what they're showing you. And it's like a film running isn't it?'

'Yeah, but I'm *in* the film though.'

Her husband knocks on the window to jog her along because she's gone over time. She burns the audio recording of my reading on a CD and hands it to me.

In the car, on the way home, the reading is playing around in my head. There was a lot that was really impressive. She described Ciaran in a way that I haven't found words for. She seemed to know him inside out. And I've no doubt that Ian Clapp was really with me. Her impression of him was uncanny. I wonder if the coincidence with the postcode of my flat was his doing! It's where my family lived when we were together so it's like a little nod from him. It was certainly reassuring when I signed the contract, and it let me know I was being supported by spirit. I've definitely got what I came for with the reading.

That whole twin thing, though. It was totally left field. When she first mentioned it I thought, *where the hell is she going with this? How is it relevant to my episodes?* It seemed to come out of nowhere. I think she might have been making it up because she didn't know what to say about my mental health problems.

Then a memory flashes through my head, confirming everything she's said. The whole twin charade in that first episode, where I folded up the sheets and then I went out into the corridor and saw more twins in the form of laundry trolleys masquerading as cots. That's what my psyche was trying to tell me. The penny drops, sending a shiver up my spine, which explodes in my head like a firework.

I *am* a twin and I wonder if it was my sister I heard tell me I was beautiful.

A dam of grief breaks free and I have to pull over because I can barely see the road for tears.

CHAPTER TWENTY SIX

Dolphin

Rebecca and I have become firm friends since my split with Ciaran. Rebecca did a shamanic practitioner course a while ago and she wants to practise some of the tools she has learnt. I'm curious to find out what my power animal is so I agree to her leading me on a journey to discover it. I'm hoping it's a bear or a wolf or something equally wild and ferocious.

Her apartment is stylish and overlooks the River Dart in town. It has unusual objects displayed like a gallery: test tubes and bugs, old wine crates for shelves and lots of her hand-thrown pottery. She's prepared a space on the floor with cushions for me to lie down on. She lights a candle and then smudges me with sage.

'I'm going to guide you with my voice and a drum. When we begin, say out loud your intention three times. "I'm going on a journey to find my power animal." The drumming will go on for about fifteen minutes and then when you hear me slow down and beat four long beats come back to your starting place. OK?'

'OK.'

'So close your eyes and speak your intention three times.'

'I'm going on a journey to find my power animal. I'm going on a journey to find my power animal. I'm going on a journey to find my power animal.'

'Let your body relax into the mat and feel supported by the earth. Find a place in the world, in your imagination, that feels very safe for you. It could be out in nature, somewhere you've been that felt really powerful.'

I take myself to a large rock by the River Dart that I usually sit on to watch the water go by. It's where we swam on the qigong camp and I felt myself being plugged into the earth by the magnetic pull of the warmed granite.

Then the drumming begins, slow at first.

'Settle yourself in your power place and have a look around you.'

The drumming speeds up, four beats a second making my brain foggy and unable to think.

'Now set off on your journey. You can travel by any means. Just let yourself be taken.'

I try to fly upwards but I don't go anywhere. Next I try the more obvious walking but again I've not moved. I feel stuck. I'm at a loss as to how to get off the power spot. I think about jumping in the river and swimming and suddenly I'm washed out to the estuary and taken in double quick time to Dingle Bay in Ireland, home to Fungi the dolphin. I went there for a holiday with Ciaran not long ago. He'd spent a year or so there and wanted to show me the place he fell in love with. I'd always wanted to go, especially to see Fungi, who I'd heard about since I was a teenager. I can't get the idea of Fungi out of my head.

Is dolphin my power animal? That's so corny and embarrassing. I hope it's not true. I don't get taken anywhere else and no other animals show up on my journey. I'm stuck in Dingle resisting the idea of having a dolphin as a spirit guide. Deep down I would love to have a dolphin as my spirit guide and when I reach that thought my eyes fill with salty tears. Maybe dolphin *is* my guide.

The fast drumming stops, banging four slower beats. I make my way back to the warm, safe rock by the river.

'You're welcome to share your journey with me if you like,' Rebecca says when I open my eyes. I tell her what happened, adding that I'm unsure if dolphin is really my power animal.

'I would trust it. Everybody experiences journeying differently. From what you've said it sounds like dolphin is your spirit animal guide.'

* * *

Some of my Shakti friends are doing the Women's Initiatory Journey. It's a year-long intensive course that cuts through unhealthy patterns of conditioned behaviour and encourages women to reconnect with each other and be mirrors for each other to rediscover their feminine power. The Shakti dance classes are a form of preparation for it and I want to join this year's group but I'm sure it will precipitate another episode so I don't sign up. I've finally learnt my lesson as any intense therapeutic work like that is sure to send me over the edge.

The women I know from the previous year's Journey speak a different language that I'm picking up gradually. I hear about the 'core wound' being 'triggered' and their 'little one' or their 'teenager' needing attention. Self-parenting is something they practise on a daily basis, to soothe the wounded parts of themselves so they don't keep acting out unconscious strategies. I'm curious about *my* core wound so I sign up to a weekend self-parenting course that a couple of Shaktis are offering. They guide us through a meditation to discover it.

'Lie down on some cushions to make yourself comfortable. Close your eyes and let go of any tension in your body. Let yourself be taken where my words lead you. You're in a house and there's a doorway to the cellar. You gently push the door open and in front of you are ten steps downwards. Walk slowly down them, one at a time. One, two, three. With each step you are going deeper underground. Four, five, six. It's dark and you can't see in front of you. Seven, eight, nine, ten. At the bottom, there's a long corridor, which you walk along. At the end, it opens out into a big cave. The cave is cold and dark and wet. Water drips from the ceiling. You creep inside making your way to the very end. There at the back of the cave is your core wound.'

A grey turd that has turned to stone lies curled up on the ground. An uncomfortable feeling makes its way through my body. My face flushes with heat and I feel nauseous. I remember this horrible sensation from my episodes: the time I flopped down by my front door when my parents came to get me; when my friend was babysitting me and

I collapsed; when I crawled under the bed and rubbed my knees raw; when I got stuck under the tree and Dad led me out. I haven't recognised this emotion before because it's been hidden away. I've done all I can to avoid feeling it lurking there in the shadows. It's why I try to be liked, why I get defensive, why I'm a perfectionist, and why I blame others. Uncovering it now, I realise most of my behaviour has been some kind of cover-up for it.

It's shame.

* * *

Marjory's predictions come true when I get a call from a TV production company in Plymouth offering me work. The film I was making for the Transition Network is finished and I've been putting my feelers out for another contract. It starts off manageably, being sent to pick up various shots that are needed in the edit for a series that's already underway, *My Tasty Travels With Lynda Bellingham*. Then word gets around that my camera work is pretty good, so my responsibilities increase. I direct Lynda on a couple of shoots, filming Concorde at Brooklands and dolphins in Cardigan Bay. It leads to more work with the same company on another series called *Storage Hoarders*. This is how it usually goes in television. If you're there you get the work but out of sight, out of mind.

The schedule is gruelling and it takes its toll on me. I'm wound up and worried about whether I've got enough footage or whether I've got the shots they need or if they'll be able to edit a sequence from them.

Roles seem to have changed within the industry. I used to be employed from the start of a programme, developing the content, being part of setting the shoots up and then going out with a crew to film before coming back to the edit suite and sitting alongside the editor. Now it's all broken up so I have nothing to do with the research or setting up the shoots. I get given a schedule, often last thing at night, for the next day telling me what I'm going to be filming: everybody's names, what they do and what they're supposed to talk about. This means I'm up late preparing and finding out where I need to be the following day. The footage is all captured digitally on cards rather than tape so I have to transfer it all onto a drive after the shoot to make space on the cards for the next day's filming. There's no time to rest after a hard day's work. I never get to see anything that I've shot because nowadays an edit producer sits with the editor creating a more efficient but factory style programme making.

I feel like a cog in a wheel and expected to operate like a machine. It takes me ages to settle to sleep at night because my head is so filled with the day just gone and anxieties for the day ahead.

For every shoot I get sent a different hire car that I have to figure out how to operate. One morning I spend ages trying to move the seat into position because it's computerised and I just can't figure it out. I shout at the car, banging on the steering wheel.

'Where the fuck is the lever to move the seat? How am I supposed to adjust the fucking seat? There must be a button somewhere. I can't fucking go anywhere without being able to reach the fucking pedals! Why the fuck have they fixed a problem that didn't exist? I fucking hate this! *Arggghhhhhh*!' I'm too stressed to enjoy driving a brand new car.

Despite this slow start, I make it to Wandsworth in good time. I'm meeting an Elizabeth Cummings who's spent thousands on storage after her husband passed away. She's been house sitting and living quite nomadically for eleven years. She describes herself as a healer and wants help to empty her storage containers so she can move on with her life.

Elizabeth greets me at the door with a warm smile. What luck that my first recce is with a like-minded soul.

'You're lucky you got me!' I tell her beaming. 'I'm a shiatsu practitioner and very sympathetic to your healing abilities. Most people in the industry will think it's a load of rubbish and mock it.'

'That's so funny! My son will love that when I tell him what you just said. You're lucky you got me!' She mimics, chuckling to herself.

We sit in the living room and a scraggy old cat slowly walks over and stands at my feet waiting for something.

'I think he wants to get into your lap.'

I help the cat up as he has little physical strength. He sits facing me and closes his eyes. He doesn't seem to want stroking.

'That's interesting. He doesn't normally like people.' Elizabeth swings her pendulum. 'He's come to give you some healing.'

'Really?'

'Did you have a cat when you were little?'

'No but this stray came into our house and had kittens in a big vase in the corridor.'

'Well, you felt really sad about having to give up the kittens but you were such a good little girl you didn't show your emotions. He's just healing that for you now.'

A huge lump comes to my throat. I did love those kitties and *really* wanted to keep them. I can almost smell their milky fur and hear their tiny meows as I remember back.

Elizabeth swings her pendulum again.

'I'm told I need to do some healing on your atlas, at the top of your spine.' The atlas is the most superior vertebra and I remember it from shiatsu. 'It needs realigning to allow the energy to flow through.' I've heard of atlas realignment. Someone offers this in Totnes and it costs a lot of money. Elizabeth closes her eyes and I wait. How is she healing me from across the other side of the room?

I'm secretly enjoying myself, but time is ticking on and we haven't talked about the filming yet. I'm supposed to be on a recce, a military term, from the word *reconnaissance*. I'm here to ascertain whether I think she'll be good in the series. How well does she express herself, and will she be able to handle the filming process, which is quite intense? The presenter, Aggie MacKenzie, and a film crew will spend a whole day with her and she'll have to go through her storage unit and decide what to keep, what to sell, and what to recycle. Not only will it be emotional, there'll be a camera in her face expecting her to be entertaining.

'Elizabeth. I'm a little anxious because I'm here to work and I haven't done any yet.'

'This *is* your work,' she responds sternly. She's right. It's no accident that my first jaunt on this series is to check out a healer. This is much more my work than the stupid format show I'm *meant* to be working on so I decide to relax and enjoy the rest of my time with her.

She's an interesting woman. She's a white South African and she and her husband were involved in the care industry in Cape Town. They pretty much started the hospice movement there. She helped people come to terms with their dying process so they could pass over more peacefully. I like her. She'll be good on the programme. She talks about a big family dining table that they all used to sit around that will be the hardest item in her storage unit to let go of. Her grief is still close to the surface. Although she communicates with her husband on the other side, she still misses him and wants him here in the flesh.

I'm with her for two hours instead of my usual one and it doesn't give me much time to get back into the centre of London to meet the next contributor. I get in the hire car, reset the sat nav and put the radio on. Ronan Keating comes on; the lyrics to 'Fires' light up my heart again and I turn the volume up.

Various people I know who have passed over come strongly to mind: those who might be lighting fires for me. My parents' next-door neighbour, Harry, worked on Concorde, where I've just directed Lynda Bellingham. He was my childhood friend's dad, the one who gave me the furry rooster during my first episode. Harry drank his way through life, working as cabin crew and then running a pub in his retirement, giving me a place to work during the holidays when I was a student. Proud of serving on Concorde, he brought his family to visist us when we were in Hong Kong, thanks to his company concessions. The life and soul of any party, he was one of those drunks who avoided destroying his life, apart from drinking himself into an early grave that is. Next, our old West African grey parrot, Peta, who I just saw—or one just like her—on the first episode of *Storage Hoarders* enters my head. My folks got her when we lived in Nigeria. A guy came around with a box full of chicks that Mum felt sorry for, so she bought the most lively looking one. Thinking she was a boy, we called her Peter. But when she was seven years old she laid an egg, so we changed the spelling to Peta. She was a perfect mimic and loved having her head stroked. She said hello when the phone rang and made the sound of the door knocking when she heard a car pulling up on the gravel outside. We thought she would live until she was seventy but she died when I was thirty. She probably wasn't suited to the English weather. Finally I think about Ian Clapp, my first boyfriend who made himself known to the medium. Bizarrely I learnt of his death in a nightclub in Hong Kong. I was out with my sister and we met a woman in the toilets who we recognised from our hometown. She was just filling us in on the news from Marple. It's uncanny how news from England made its way across the world to us like that. Well before the internet, with no social media, we wouldn't have found out about it otherwise.

I let through all the grief I held back during the cat healing, moved by all these people from my past, in my mind or in spirit, lighting the way home.

CHAPTER TWENTY SEVEN

Retreat

I t's been over eighteenth months since I left Ciaran. We've managed to make it through the divorce proceedings without any costly solicitors. The decree nisi has come through so we've got six weeks to change our minds before it's final. I'm secretly hoping Ciaran will show up with all the right words and claim me as his forever. But that's just hanging on to a fairytale.

To mark the occasion I invite a few friends around for a divorce ritual. We sit in my conservatory living room, spilling over onto cushions on the floor to watch two videos. One is a music video I made to go with a song Ciaran wrote for my fortieth birthday. Rachael, the singer-songwriter who rented an office space in our house, put some music to it and sang it for him at my party. I remember making a joke when she performed it about wondering why they were spending so much time together. They hadn't been spending a lot of time together but I didn't realise at the time how prophetic that joke was. I knew he fancied her. Everybody does. She's such a goddess.

'Wow what an honouring! He really got you didn't he?' Andrea concludes when the song has finished. She has never met Ciaran and I experience a sudden pang for him. I respect Andrea. She's managed to get a space at the local GP surgery to do her weird and wonderful healing work. She's part of the crowd of women I've surrounded myself with since Ciaran and I separated.

The other video is the one I edited of our wedding. I love watching it. I look so serene at the registry office. I don't really want our marriage to be over but I have to accept that it is. There was a moment when we discussed getting back together but it didn't feel right. We tiptoed around it, neither of us showing our true feelings, protecting our pain. But ultimately we hadn't resolved anything so getting back together wasn't going to solve our problems. Watching us get married brings up more sadness. I wipe the tears from my eyes before leading us into the next part of the wet November evening.

Carrying a black, heart-shaped velvet box with my wedding ring inside, we form a procession in silence, like a funeral wake. It's not far to walk around the corner to the cemetery. I find a small patch of ground, next to a stone wall, just under a beech tree. Forming a circle we dance down into our depths and spontaneously sing a random cacophony of individual notes that make up a harmonious but haunting sound.

I dig a shallow grave with a trowel and lay the 'coffin' gently in the bottom, smoothing the scattered earth back over the top. We all pat it down in turn, stamping our feet like a rain dance, even though it's already raining.

* * *

The founder of the Spiritual Crisis Network, Catherine Lucas, has a book out, *In Case of Spiritual Emergency*. She's included some contributions from people who've been through a spiritual crisis and I'm one of them. I order ten copies and hand them out to my close friends, inviting them to support me through my next episode. They all want to help. I now have a team of ten women on hand just in case.

I particularly relish the chapter on modern mystics. Eckhart Tolle features in it as does Amma, the hugging saint. Amma travels the world, hugging thousands of people at a time. Before she became the guru figure she is today, she went through her own process of spiritual emergency. She was born in a small fishing village in Kerala, in southern India, in 1953. Like Cinderella, her family treated her like a servant. She spent hours in prayer, asking Krishna to reveal himself to her. As she got older, she would disappear into altered states of consciousness as she merged into deep spiritual rapture with Him. Her family thought she had schizophrenia as she became unable to look after herself in these states. She experienced a terrific heat in her body, typical of the rising Kundalini energy, and would bury herself in the earth. I feel honoured to be counted alongside these two giants of the New Age.

What might I become if I manage to go through my episodes without the interference of the psychiatric system closing me down with antipsychotics?

* * *

Andrea's having another darkness and silence retreat for the winter solstice. I went last year and it was a good way to mark the turning point of the year. The decree absolute arrived in the post this morning so I take it with me to put on the altar. The end of my marriage *and* the end of 2012. The Mayans believe it's the end of a phase in our history and it's definitely the end of a phase in my personal history.

As the sun is setting, we gather in Andrea's living room and watch the flames of a fire, our only light, flickering in the hearth. From this moment on we won't speak until tomorrow. We do communicate but just through our faces, our actions, and our energy.

The quiet feels more bearable than last year, when I was stuck with a head full of negative thoughts, feeling the discomfort and weirdness of what we were doing. But this year it's easier. In fact it's quite welcome. I usually talk far too much, mostly out of nervousness. Not speaking is allowing me to settle more deeply into myself, even though I'm with other people.

We're sprawled around the room, taking up all the available spaces: Andrea is near the fire, tending it like a loving mother; Natasha, a Polish woman whose translucent skin makes her seem delicate, has her legs dangling casually over the side of the armchair; Lisa is on the other armchair, probably relieved everyone is now as quiet as she; Angela sits rigidly upright and cross-legged in meditation; Tanja, the enemy I keep close, is lying on the couch; while I'm on the floor, leaning against the arm of the sofa. Occasionally someone fidgets to find a new position. Shadows flicker around the room from the light cast by the fire. We all stare incessantly at it, watching the only entertainment available. The orange flames curl and lap around the wood. Our faces are dimly lit but our pupils shine like big, black saucers.

Two flames lick around a round log, turning different colours of orange, red, purple, and pink. Symmetrically mirroring each other, they loop over the wood and meet in the middle forming a perfect heart shape. It burns like this for at least a minute and we all see it, pointing, gawping, and delighted by the magic. We're probably all thinking a similar thing: spirit is sending us love.

We nest down early for the night as there's little else to do. The lack of stimulation is making us all feel our deep, winter tiredness. I head upstairs to crash in one of the kid's beds. I'm not sure where Andrea's children are but they're staying elsewhere so we can all be here in silence.

I wake just before dawn and gather up the others to join me for the sunrise. It's a hilly part of the world so finding a clear view is tricky. We can't agree on the best place and walk around the fields before ending up back in Andrea's back garden. The others coo at the sunrise in the distance but I'm too short to see over the high fence. Tucked in the corner and surrounded by weeds is a trampoline. It gives me an idea. I bounce on it and as I reach the full height of the upwards spring, I see the sun sitting on the horizon. I hover in the air for the shortest time but long enough to feel a sunbeam reach out and kiss my face. Multicoloured tentacles of light magnetise towards me and caress my cheek, a beautiful morning greeting.

Then Andrea leads the way down to the river, through the pine wood of Huxham's Cross. She detours off the muddy path and into the dark belly of the forest. All holding hands in an unbroken line, Andrea takes us to a den. Someone has made a huge hideout, sunk into the ground and covered over with branches. The way winds around, just high enough to bend down in. The energy in Lisa's hand starts to quiver. What is she so afraid of? The path drops down a step, which slows us all down, making us all wait for each woman behind to find her way. Around another corner and the den continues on. It's total darkness, a labyrinth into the heart of the earth. One by one we emerge out of the other side and into the daylight.

We pick up the track further down and follow it to the edge of the wood. It opens out onto a muddy field. My feet slip beneath me and I don't bother trying to prevent a fall. It's easier to just go with it, letting my hands catch my weight. Andrea turns and smiles at me with a mischievous look in her eyes. I reach up and wipe her face with the sticky clay. She grins and scoops up some earth onto her finger and draws some lines on my face. It sets off a chain reaction in the others.

We look like feral creatures, a tribe of wild sisters, initiated by the land herself.

The rest of the way I hold tightly onto the stone in my pocket, smoothing it with my thumb. We've each picked one from a bag that Andrea gathered earlier for the occasion. She's the main organiser, and is leading the proceedings.

The River Dart is dangerously high, covering the pebble beach that people hang out on in the summer. The bank where you can normally climb down is now covered in water. It's flowing fast too. Andrea stops and waits for us all to circle around.

'I let go of fear,' she calls out loudly, holding her pebble up in the air. 'I let go of playing small. I let go of men who no longer serve me.' She runs through a long list and then hurtles the stone into the river. Each in turn calls out all the things she wants to give up in her life: distractions, addictions, beliefs, behaviours. Any way that any of us is avoiding being the shining lights that we are is named, and offered to the river.

Then Andrea strips off and dunks in the freezing water. Lisa, too, takes her clothes off and steps into the cold. She may be afraid of the dark but she's certainly not bothered by temperature. I wouldn't even go naked in this December chill, let alone into these icy waters.

Lisa loses her footing and calls out as the river tries to pull her downstream. Andrea grabs her and forms a chain with others to heave her out onto the bank.

All dried off, we return to the house and break the silence. Sitting in a circle beside the fire, we share words. When I speak, I feel like I'm reaching down into a black void. I don't know what I'm going to say until the words come out, as if standing before an abyss and taking a step anyway. I have to wait on the threshold for the next sentence to come. It doesn't feel like it's coming from my brain but through my body, my womb perhaps. And my womb is picking it up from somewhere else.

I hear myself talking about the number of people around the world who are waking up at this time: people who are seeing what we're doing to the planet and trying to change things. Many are struggling to be part of a world that doesn't care that it's destroying the precious ecosystems that are vital for our survival. Whatever I say is having an impact because Tanja, sitting next to me, is weeping. I keep on, delivering this apparently channelled message and enjoying the freedom from fear that usually grips me when I enter the unknown.

With the silence broken, we gather around the kitchen table to share food. There's a buzz between us that wasn't there before, of people who know each other really well, because of a shared experience: a feeling of community. And in my heart there's another buzz: of a bee nuzzling into a flower and feeding on the sweet nectar.

'I'm really drawn to you,' Natasha says to me in her Polish drawl, her eyelids closing slowly in their usual, sensual way.

'Yes. I feel a lovely buzz in my heart. That's probably what you're attracted to.' As soon as I've said it I tense up. Feeling this good means another episode is on its way.

CHAPTER TWENTY EIGHT

Journeying

I make my way into town on foot, detouring slightly to visit Leech-well, a healing spring where lepers used to bathe. Nowadays hip-pies treat it as a sacred site, tying ribbons or leaving crystals and flowers around the barred entrance. The water that runs off the hills and into this well is actually full of pesticides.

I pause at the opening in the rock, breathing the cold air and listen-ing to the trickling of the water landing in the stone troughs beneath the spouts. I take a deep and conscious breath in to receive the healing energies, if there are any. A sudden cold and sharp wind slams into my lower belly.

What the fuck was that?

I continue my way down the path, sheltered on either side by high walls, built to hide the lepers from the rich townsfolk of Totnes.

The Civic Hall is packed and dark. The winter solstice 5Rhythms event is always well attended. People dress up as if it's New Year's Eve. It attracts lots of newcomers and people who only come to the class intermittently. I've been going every Monday, to connect with myself and the community for a while now. I find it quite challenging and have to get past my judgements of everyone before I can actually enjoy it.

Marianne, another Shakti, who I don't really hang out with, greets me as I hang up my coat.

'Can I have a hug?'

'Why?' I ask, hoping she'll leave me alone. I just want to be in my own space.

'Something shocking just happened,' she says pitifully, opening her arms and making her way towards me like a little girl needing her mother. I go through the hugging motions, feeling no sympathy. Hugs are expected in Totnes, like a human right.

'What is it that you can't take in Marianne?' I ask her, with our arms still around each other. I know from shiatsu that shock is what happens when we're not able to assimilate. 'What is it that you don't want to let in, Marianne? Focus on that, and welcome it.' Something seeps out of my lower belly and moves into hers. Then she lets go of me and skips away merrily. Whatever it was that slammed into me has found a new host.

The dance floor is crowded and I don't feel like connecting with anyone. Everyone looks slightly insane to me. I clock one person who looks so full of self-loathing his eyes are darting about, shiftily avoiding eye contact. Another is in that 'Totnes love-bubble' kind of high state, smiling inanely at anyone who will look. I face the wall, hoping to shut them all out. I'm feeling deep down, shamanic, and not in the mood for social niceties.

A guy leaps behind me, stopping to wriggle his back against mine. It feels like a theft. I don't see who it is but I'm pretty sure I know. I'm guessing it's the French guy who's been trying to meet up with me. We met at a party I went to after my divorce ritual.

'What is it that you want me to know about you?' he had asked me, leaning forwards and glaring into my eyes as if I was the goddess herself.

'I've just come from my divorce ritual.' I paused, waiting for his response, but there wasn't one. Well, not verbal anyhow. He let out an exaggerated sigh in the way Totnes people do, as if to say, 'I hear you, and resonate with you.' After a long silence, I thought to ask him the same question. At first he was insecure that his answer wouldn't be as good as mine and then he said,

'I want you to know that I aspire to peace and love.' He's been messaging me to arrange a meeting but luckily our texts didn't get through.

I shake him off and try to concentrate on the dance. I see Angela across the room so I head over to see how she is after the retreat. She's also feeling ultra-sensitive to everybody's energy.

'You know, Emma, before I came, I gave myself permission to leave if I felt it was too much.'

'Thanks, Angela. That's a good idea. I think I'm going to go. Enjoy the rest of your evening.'

I catch the Frenchman's eye as I make my way towards the exit. He looks at me questioningly, like a lost puppy. I lift my hand to say a polite farewell and leave without smiling.

* * *

Apocalyptic floods hit the West Country disrupting traffic and preventing trains from departing. We're advised not to travel unless we absolutely have to. The train I'm booked on to go up north for Christmas is so delayed it will mean missing my connection in Birmingham and sleeping on the platform until the next one leaves in the morning. I'm quietly relieved. I don't think travelling is a good idea at the moment. I'm trying to stay as grounded as possible to ride this out without having to go into hospital.

I hunker down on the sofa, covered in blankets, expecting the worst. I remember the psychic medium Marjory's advice to stop being the viewer and start asking questions.

'What's going on?' I say in my head. 'Who's here?'

A big hornet buzzes on the far wall, lifts off and flies towards my bookshelf. It lands on a paperback. *The Magdalene Manuscript* is a channelled book, recounting the adventures of Mary Magdalene and Jesus Christ. It claims they were tantric lovers and practised sexual alchemy to prepare him for his role as spiritual leader.

'If you're the Magdalene, show me a miracle.' Something tells me to look at the conservatory door that opens onto the back garden. Raindrops slide down the pane of glass. One is stationary, suspended as if defying gravity. Is that a miracle? I think about filming it but then realise no one would believe videos these days. I could have made it happen through special effects. And anyway, I'm sure blobs of water have to be a certain weight before they start sliding downwards. Maybe it hasn't reached its saturation point. If it were moving upwards I'd be more inclined to believe it was a miracle.

'So what's this all about?'

The answer that comes to me is, 'Finding God'.

'And what's the point of that?'

No answer arrives. I imagine what a dull world it would be if we were all enlightened and communing with God. What would be the point, then? And anyway, I read recently in one of Carlos Castaneda's books that it turns out that God is just a big eagle who sucks us back into itself when we die. I don't like the sound of that.

'How do I know God is the good guy?' Again, no answer.

I grab my house keys and put them in my coat pocket, then slip my mobile in the other. I push up my umbrella and brace myself against the rain.

I always bump into people at the Happy Apple. It's a ten o'clock shop that sells healthy organic foods as well as the usual cigarettes and alcohol. I've never seen my shiatsu practitioner, Nick Turner, here before. He's standing by the fruit and veg in the alleyway.

'Hi, Nick. How are you?'

'Hello, Emma. I'm a little busy. I've got the family over for Christmas. What about you?'

I want to tell him that it's synchronicity that I should meet him here because I'm slipping into another episode. During a shiatsu session with him, he disclosed that he'd been through a similar awakening in his life in his thirties and he was terrified he was losing his mind. He said it by way of offering to support me in the future. I wasn't sure if he meant outside the sessions or just as a practitioner. I'm dying to ask him if he'll come and help me.

'I'm OK. I've just come back from a darkness and silence retreat so I feel a bit strange.'

'Well, I'll be around over the holidays if you need me.'

'Thanks, Nick.'

I feel a sense of relief and feel looked-after, bumping into Nick like that. I don't think it's an accident that we were at the same place at the same time. Of all the people I know in this town, he's probably the only one who could give me some useful professional help.

When I get home, my phone isn't in my pocket. When did I last have it? I responded to a text on the way into Totnes. I retrace my steps back to the same spot where I took it out of my pocket, just near the end of the lane, but it's nowhere to be seen, so I rush home and call my network provider.

'I need to report a lost phone.'

'When did you lose it?'

'Just earlier today. I know it sounds crazy but it just popped out of the universe. It was in my pocket, and now it's not.'

'What do you want me to do?

'Well, put a stop on it until it reappears.'

'OK. Let us know if you find it.'

I'm full of energy that's swirling around my body desperate to go somewhere but I don't know what to do with it. I call Rebecca, my shamanic practitioner friend, to see if I can go round to hers. We had a bit of a falling out recently and haven't really sorted things out properly yet. It was all because I couldn't keep my mouth shut in an email. I'd mentioned I was thinking about doing the Women's Initiatory Journey. Rebecca responded with a big 'No'. I replied that I preferred it if my friends would trust me to make my own decisions. That triggered her, and she went a bit crazy on the phone. I felt freaked out and, although I wanted to sort it out, I was too afraid to meet up. That was a couple of weeks ago.

Rebecca has her mother staying but she says it's fine to come around. She's not that well and is feeling pretty wiped out. I don't want a big heavy conversation but I do feel like reconnecting with her. She looks a little bleary-eyed when she opens the door to me. Her mum sits quietly reading, and lifts her head up briefly to say 'Hi'. Rebecca lies down on the sofa and I kneel on the floor beside her.

'I'm full of healing energy after the winter solstice retreat.'

'I'm wiped out and just want to sleep all the time.'

'Do you mind if I put my hand on you?'

'Sure. Go ahead.' I've given Rebecca shiatsu treatments before so I don't think it's such a strange thing to do. I place my palm on her leg and a load of energy leaves my body and flows into her.

'Does that feel OK?'

'Yes. It's warm.'

'Are you open to having a conversation about what happened?'

'No,' Rebecca replies abruptly.

Her snappiness stops me in my tracks. I don't react but instead wait, feeling the discomfort of the moment until it passes. I sit for what feels like an age, with nothing useful to say. Eventually a different question pops into my head.

'Are you open to *me*?'

'Oh, yes!' she says, warmly, so I relax.

'Can you feel all the energy coming out of my hand?'

'Yes.'

'It feels better for it to have somewhere to go.'

Then we return to a silence. I continue with the holding until I sense it's finished then I wish them both a happy Christmas and leave.

That night I can't get to sleep and it sends me into a spin of worry. Sleeping is crucial. I'm convinced it's what tipped me over in the first episode. I think I ended up going into a waking dream state because of the deprivation. As if my brain so needed to dream, that it went ahead and did it anyway, even though I was awake.

What if Rebecca is doing all the sleeping for me? Maybe that's why she's so wiped out. She's feeling the tiredness that I can't feel. I *must* get to sleep *so* Rebecca can be more awake. But I *can't*. Maybe I have to kill myself so that Rebecca can have more energy. Now that sounds a bit odd, and might not be true. I don't want to kill myself. I will if I have to, but maybe I should check it out with someone else first.

'Magda?' Magda is one of the ten women on my care team. I know her from Shakti dancing and she assists Isabella with the classes sometimes.

'Hi Emma. How are you?'

'Can I do a reality check with you?'

'Sure. Go ahead.'

'I'm having some strange thoughts. I can't get to sleep and that's usually a sign that something is wrong. I was thinking that my not being able to sleep means that my friend Rebecca is sleeping for me. Is that your reality?'

'That's not my reality.'

'OK. Thanks, Magda,' and I hang up and settle back down in bed.

My flat has been converted from a house into two apartments. My bedroom was originally a living room. The wardrobe blocks off a door that's no longer in use, which opens into the hall by the front door. If I went through the back of it I'd end up on the street, like in *The Lion, the Witch and the Wardrobe*. It's totally fitting given that Totnes is twinned with Narnia. It's why I moved here: so that people would accept my episodes as spiritual rather than freak out that I'm crazy.

The image of a dolphin appears in my head. The left side of its face is nestled snugly into the left side of mine, our eyes perfectly lined up. It's grey blue wet skin, permanently smiling mouth, and shiny eyes feel friendly and supportive. Through some strange transfer of knowledge, it tells me not to worry. It tells me that it will help me sleep, like a dolphin. Dolphins have the ability to rest each hemisphere of their brain separately because they have to stay conscious in order to breathe. If they fall asleep they die so they've evolved to have only half of their brain sleep at a time.

The lower right hand side of my head goes fuzzy, a numbness. It's like this for ages and then another part of my brain goes numb. I follow it all night, trusting that it's my power animal helping me. My brain is sleeping, one cortex at a time and maybe that's enough. It takes the pressure off me worrying about not sleeping, anyhow.

In the morning I'm full of energy again, but not because it's Christmas Day. I put my wellies on to head out over the fields behind my house for my usual morning walk. The rain has abated so I reach for my red wool coat, the one I was wearing when I first met Ciaran. Inside the pocket I find my mobile. How odd. I definitely put it in my brown, waxed cotton jacket. How the hell did it get into *this* pocket? Maybe it's the miracle I asked for.

I call up my service provider again to explain that my phone has popped back into the universe via a different coat pocket. They probably think I just lost track of it but I don't care. I don't need them to believe me, as long as they take the block off it.

The path through the woods is extra muddy, sucking at my boots. The stream is full but it's still possible to wade through. At least I don't have to worry about cows chasing me. They're kept off the fields in the winter so I walk along the ridge to my favourite oak tree.

'Hello, Oak,' I greet it, stepping around its exposed roots, stroking the jagged bark. Stopping where I started, I lean back and rest against the trunk. The energy drains out of my head and into the tree. All of the racing, full, pumping energy goes, leaving my brain feeling clearer, empty, and spacious so I feel normal again.

I continue on my way, wading along a green lane that's deep in water. I go through the woods and over the fields, winding my way indirectly towards Dartington. I wonder about miracles and what they actually are. I think our minds are more powerful than any of us truly know. A miracle is just someone being so convinced of an outcome that it actually comes about. But with something that doesn't seem possible, like making the blind see.

I was fascinated by the study of perception in my psychology degree. How our consciousness happens is one of the great remaining mysteries of science. It is a kind of controlled hallucination happening through, and because of, our bodies. Perception, figuring what's out there in the world, is informed guesswork based on the signals received from our senses. There are lots of visual illusions that demonstrate how our brains don't see reality accurately. Two circles with the exact same diameter look completely different depending on the size of the circles that surround them: smaller circles make the inner one look larger; larger circles make the inner one look smaller. We see wrongly and the world we see comes from the inside out as much as the outside in. Our brains use prior expectations to construct reality.

Perception is really just a controlled hallucination. We're all hallucinating all the time and when we agree on it, we call it 'reality'. We mostly take for granted our experience of having a bodily self, for example. We can't imagine mistaking anything else for it, or our bodies for anything else. But there's something called the rubber hand illusion that proves otherwise. The subject's real hand is hidden from view while a fake hand is put in front of them. Both are stroked simultaneously, which leads the person to think that the fake hand is in fact part of their body. When the experimenter suddenly stabs the fake rubber hand with a knife, the subject instinctively pulls their own hand away.

Just before my finals, I made the arguably unwise decision to take LSD. I had broken my leg, having fallen off a rock that I was climbing while stoned, and a friend suggested an acid trip to cheer me up. As soon as I felt the effects taking place, I noticed 'The Future Sound of London' record sleeve in the corner of the room. The weird pixelated face on the cover was moving. I stared at it wondering what else I could achieve with my mind if I could make this picture become animated. With some unknown power of perception and a little help from the drug, but initiated entirely by my desire, thoughts, and will power, my gaze pulled on the image to stretch the effects wider until the whole room was pixelated. I scared myself silly and just as easily switched the whole thing off, preferring to huddle on the sofa until the effects of the acid had worn off.

I reach Elizabeth's house, another Shakti, where I've been for ceremonies and Shakti dancing and evenings of music performance and storytelling. Her living room is filled with sheepskin rugs and shamanic objects and pictures on the wall. As I walk past, I feel a massive heart-shaped pumping ball of energy leap out of her house towards me.

Further down the lane, just before my turn-off, three women walk ahead of me in the same direction. One of them is Shelly, the woman who made me realise I should have told Ciaran three times that I wasn't enjoying myself on the first night. I slow down so as not to overtake them, but they stop just as they get to the junction that I'll be turning at.

'It's you! Happy Christmas,' Shelly says, giving me a hug, once I've caught them up.

'Yes. Happy Christmas.'

'We're all going back to my friend's for a meal. If you're on your own, would you like to join us?'

'I think I need to be alone.' I can't imagine being able to make conversation at a stranger's house.

Shelly can sense I'm not myself and looks into my eyes, really close up, tuning into me. I can feel some energy spinning in my eyes as she holds my gaze.

'Journeying,' she says.

'Yes.' I break eye contact and turn off onto the dirt track. 'My house is this way,' I say pointing down the lane and then wave.

The people around here are very different from anywhere else I've lived. They speak a different language and they have strong spiritual beliefs. Some of them are lost, or damaged, or sick, or all three, but they're all searching for connection and community. I moved here so I would be around people who shared my spiritual take on things and wouldn't see me as psychotic. Shelly's one word, 'journeying', reassures me that I'm OK. I'm on a shamanic kind of journey and it can only be done alone. I don't know what I'll find or how to navigate properly but I know I've got ten women who are willing to help me out if I need it. They don't think I'm crazy. Just sensitive, and open, and easily transported to other realms.

I head back over the stream, through the woods, under the railway, and back onto Smithfields, the cul-de-sac where I live. Flames are flickering out of the chimney of one of the houses. A woman across the road panics, calling her husband to come and have a look. He rushes out just as someone from the house that's on fire appears in the garden.

'It's OK. We've got it under control,' he says. 'It's just the chimney.'

There's a general feeling of high drama but I walk through the scene serenely, like it's a film set, calm in the knowledge that it is all being taken care of. No flutter of fear tickles my solar plexus, where I would normally sense even the slightest danger.

When I get home I put some music on. Grimes's *Visions* is a strange mix of electronic beats and incoherent singing. I recently bought it from Drift Records, finding it on their list of top 100 albums of 2012. It reminds me of a cross between the Cocteau Twins and Strawberry Switchblade. It has quite a prominent baseline, floaty synthesiser, and eerie, high vocals. When the beats kick in, I dance around the kitchen, flinging my arms out and jiggling my head chaotically to the music. I'm full of energy again, which I shake out, sending shivers up my spine and through my head.

A large mirror leans against the wall, resting on the radiator. I've not bothered hanging it up properly since I moved in because it's just too big and heavy to handle on my own. I stand up close to it swaying to the music, staring right into my eyes, my large black pupils shining back at me. I widen my attention to include both eyes equally with my focus somewhere between them. Keeping my head straight forwards, I turn my body left and right to the music, with my knees bent and my feet firmly rooted to the spot.

I keep staring deep into my reflection. My hair hangs straight down either side of my face. Then my features are gone and there's nothing there but a black hole where my face should be.

I call some friends and let them know I'm in Amber and I think it's probably best if they're in regular contact with me, to make sure I'm OK. I ask Shilpa to come round and she sounds overjoyed, like she's been handpicked out of thousands. Shilpa is my love addict friend and we sit at the kitchen table and watch a candle burning. I've not been using lights for the past three weeks, preferring instead to take in the full darkness of winter. The conversation is slow and I pick up on every word, wanting to be precise and noticing how so much of our verbal communication is based on habit of expression. Quite a Zen-like dialogue takes place between us. Shilpa has just come back from a meditation retreat and I can tell she's still in that zone. It's just the kind of spiritual calm I need right now.

I hold my hands out cupping either side of the flame but I don't feel any heat from it. It should be too hot to handle but it has an almost cold feeling to it. Shilpa takes a turn and she's surprised she only lasts a couple of seconds.

'Ooooh it's hot,' she squeals quickly pulling her hands away. It *should* be hot with hands that close. I try again. My palms must be only an inch away from the burning flame but it still feels cool. I've no idea what I'm doing, but for some reason I'm not getting burned.

I watch a thick shimmer of energy rise from the flame and join the energy from my palms, like the heat haze from a hot road. I can't normally see energy and this pale, liquid gold is not unlike the ribbon I saw coming from below my belly button. It's beautiful.

Lisa and Natasha from the darkness and silence retreat are my next visitors and come round together. Half of the women on my care team are away, so I've only got five of them to help me. I'm not sure if it will be enough, given it's the Christmas holidays and they've all got other plans.

I suggest they give me a shiatsu treatment to help ground me but neither of them have a clue where to start.

'I'll guide you.' I lie down on the bed and they sit either side of me. 'Put your palms somewhere on my body, anywhere it doesn't really matter. And then lean all your weight onto me.'

The mattress springs absorb most of the pressure so I just end up sinking down into it. Natasha's waif-like frame means there's little substance behind her touch.

'It's not working,' I say, giving up. 'Let's do some of your movement medicine instead.' Lisa has trained in a form of dance that I'm curious about. It's helped her a lot and I've seen a visible difference in her. A huge weight seems to have lifted from her in the last year or so. Standing side by side in the living room, I'm amused by our extreme height difference. Lisa must be six foot and stands like a giant in comparison to me. She speaks some instructions that I internally pick apart. She has a way of speaking which is quite stilted, like she's editing everything she says. I can tell she's uncomfortable being in charge, giving directions and guidance. Rather than just tell me what to do, she says it like an optional invitation. I half-heartedly follow along, feeling mischievous and wishing she would be more assertive.

Lisa's features look part-animal, part-human. Her ears are poking out of her dark, wild, unwashed long hair. Her teeth are sharp and darkened at the edges. Her clothes are crinkled with lots of layers swamping her.

'You look like a creature from *Lord of the Rings* or something.' I burst out laughing.

Lisa laughs too but I can tell she's a little frustrated that I'm not joining in properly. Although she's shying away from being the teacher, she still wants to be in control.

I look over at Natasha who also looks like a caricature of herself. Her pointy ears are like pixies' and her pale skin like a fairy's.

'You're so elfin Natasha! You're like a little pixie.' I fall about laughing at both of them.

We give up on the movement medicine.

Natasha has to go to work but Lisa stays behind and we get out some art materials. She sits at the head of the kitchen table and runs her finger along the pencils before picking out a brown one. On a large piece of paper, she outlines the trunk and branches of a tree, her mouth twisting with concentration and the faint sound of frustration on her breath. I can tell she doesn't really want to be here. Her son is away at his dad's, leaving her a few precious days to herself, and she hadn't planned on spending them with me.

Someone must have called the GP because a Dr Andrews comes round to check up on me. He gives me a sleeping tablet and says I should be OK for the night on my own, but Lisa stays over on my sofa bed anyway, feeling overly responsible.

In the morning Nicky takes over from Lisa. I've known Nicky for over sixteen years and met her through Ella before my first episode. I liked Nicky as soon as I met her. She's sincere and trustworthy compared to the other friends I had at the time. We ended up going on a scuba-diving holiday together in Egypt, even though we hardly knew each other. Our paths in life keep crossing and we share a lot in common: we both worked in television in Bristol; we both did the same shiatsu course; we've both moved to Totnes; and we've both recently divorced.

We head out for a morning walk through a communal garden that leads into an orchard where there's a path through a little wood. Maple trees line the footpath and I ask Nicky how she would frame the view, if she was filming it, so that the trees go out of focus in the distance. She has a good eye, and composes a better shot than I do. We play around with the perspective, Nicky making her thumb and forefingers into a rectangle shape to show me how she would set up the camera.

We continue along the track before stopping again to take a closer look at one of the trees. Its orange bark is shining in the wet. We place our hands around it as if we're giving it a shiatsu. A huge whoosh of water swirls inside it, beneath the level of the ground. It's like the tree is hollowed out, like a didgeridoo and the groundwater is sloshing around inside, like the slow spin cycle of a washing machine slapping against the drum.

'Did you feel that?'

'Yes,' Nicky affirms.

'Wow. That's amazing. There must be so much water in there.'

'She's so beautiful,' Nicky says.

'How do you know it's a she?' I ask.

'I don't.'

Nicky lets me know that she's spoken to Melissa who says I'm welcome to stay at her house any time I like, but it feels too imposing. I don't want to take my weirdness into their family festivities. It also feels far too kind an offer to accept.

Back home and alone again, I collapse with that awful feeling in my stomach that I now know to be shame. It's always at this point that people feel they can't handle taking care of me any more. Sure enough the Crisis Team is called and Rebecca, Natasha, and Nicky gather in my kitchen for a meeting to discuss what we're going to do. I recognise Mia Carter from my last episode but Ben is new to me. He's short with a full ginger beard and soft voice.

The meeting seems to take ages and we keep going round in circles. The Crisis Team's role is to try to keep me out of hospital. I have insight and haven't lost my ego, so to them it probably looks like I could be safe to stay at home. I'm clear I would feel better if there was someone with me at all times and my friends are clear that they've reached their limits. I don't know why Mia and Ben are taking so long to agree to admit me to hospital.

Nicky is leaning against the kitchen unit with one foot up, locked against her thigh, like a stork. She seems a little tense with her arms folded and her eyes darting about. Rebecca is sitting on the kitchen surface visibly agitated.

'Can I just say something?' Rebecca asks looking briefly over to me and then back to Mia and Ben. 'Emma came round to my house the other day and she was behaving very strangely.'

I'm annoyed because yes, granted, I was a little odd, but only because she's not used to me being like this. In this state, I feel more authentic than I normally do and don't feel the need to cover up awkward social moments with my usual nervous talking. I was very calm when I went round to her flat and navigated a very difficult moment when she snapped at me. There's really no need to add to the reasons why she thinks I should be put into hospital, as I'm not denying my need for support. But mostly I don't like that she's using the incident when I put my healing hands on her as evidence against me. She's probably worried that the Crisis Team might insist I stay home, but I feel a deep sense of betrayal. The only reason we're discussing whether I should go into hospital is because my friends have reached the limits of their ability to care. It's not a question of how 'crazy' I am, but whether I can be supported at home. I think we should be talking about that, and not how odd my behaviour has been.

It's decided. Ben will drive me to Torbay Hospital where I can be admitted. Nicky cries as she says her farewells. It seems over the top, like an anxious mother.

'Why are you crying, Nicky?' I ask her baffled by her tears.

'Because I love you, Emma.'

Not enough to keep me out of hospital, though, I think to myself.

CHAPTER TWENTY NINE

Imprisonment

Ben drives us carefully through the busy holiday traffic, to the
Haytor Unit.
'You're a good driver.'
'Thanks.'
'Where are you from, Ben?'
'I'm a Devon boy. Born and bred.'
'I couldn't place your accent. It sounds a little West Country but it's
got clipped around the edges.'
'Yeah. I moved away for uni and travel, but I came back.'
'Ah! That's why. Have you always done this kind of work?'
'No! I used to be a Buddhist monk.'
'Really? That's why you're so calm, then.'
'Your friends seemed a little tense.'
'You noticed ...'
'One of them seemed a bit angry.'
'Yes, she was. I think they were worried you weren't going to take
me off their hands.'
Ben walks me into the psychiatric unit and tells me to sit by the door
while he goes off to liaise with the staff. It's not the same ward as last
time. Oak Ward, downstairs, has closed due to NHS cuts.

Organ music is playing loud enough for everyone on the ward to hear. I'm not sure where it's coming from. An old Wurlitzer pipes a Victorian circus theme. A most ironic welcome, which goes straight to my adrenals. There's probably a logical explanation for it. Probably the Radio Two programme *The Organist Entertains*, but I fall through a completely different trapdoor of thought.

I picture my deceased granddad, who used to play the instrument for a living, in another room on the ward, plonking away on the keyboard. All my grandparents are with him, ghosts watching over my arrival, tempting me to come in and take one of the lonely patients as a partner and join the dance. You'd think the staff would turn it off. Or down, at least.

I wait for what feels like an age before Ben comes back and hands me over to a member of staff who takes me to a small office. He puts a form in front of me and asks me to sign it. I'm not sure what I'm being asked to put my signature to so I read through the whole thing slowly. It's some kind of legal document and I think I should probably have an advocate or a solicitor present to explain it to me but I can't be bothered. It mentions something about the hospital having the right to film me. I don't object. The footage might be useful for a documentary one day.

A healthcare assistant, or whatever she is, walks me to my room, a big wad of keys jangling off her belt. She empties my bag out onto the bed, one item at a time, probably checking for anything I might use to top myself with. She lifts out the book that I'm currently reading, *The Hidden Spirituality of Men*, and tuts disapprovingly, as if to say, 'Don't bring your spiritual crap in here.' She puts it down quickly, like she's trying to avoid catching a terrible disease. Then she counts my money and writes down the amount on her form, asking if I want to keep my valuables safely locked away until I leave.

'No, thanks.'

Once she's gone, I put my clothes away wondering why they bother with a wardrobe when they don't provide any coathangers. I wouldn't even know how to kill myself with one if I wanted to. Perhaps if we weren't treated like prisoners, fewer people would want to find such a drastic way out.

Every two hours, during the night, footsteps sound along the corridor outside my room. A flash of light then appears through a little viewing window in the door followed by a pause for two seconds while the torch shines in my eyes. Then the footsteps again, this time moving away. It's a suicide watch and they're checking I'm still breathing.

The spotlight, like a searchlight hunting for criminals, triggers a past-life trauma or something. I'm escaping from Poland, I think, in a boat, with a baby. Mixed in with this is me having to dance at some kind of peep show. I writhe around feigning sexual allure, in order to stay alive. I don't want to be killed so I'd better do as expected. Sweaty fat men leer at me. One in particular has the best seat in the house. The fucking devil again.

I know the male staff are just doing the rounds, but why are they allowed onto a female ward? It's like they're taking it in turns, passing the torch round to peep in my door and watch me in bed, the horizontal pole dancer.

At one point the door opens and two people walk in. One of them appears to be the Shakti who was roaring at me at the summer solstice dance before my last episode. How can that be? She looks real enough, but I can't tell how solid she is. They stand side by side looking at me, whispering to each other. Then she barks at me.

'Don't stay 'ere Em.'

She sounds disappointed that I'm back in this place. They stand there for a few more minutes, whispering to each other and then leave without saying goodbye. I'm not sure if they were spirits, or staff that are triggering another past-life flashback.

By morning I realise it's a mistake coming here. I would be better off on my own at home. I pack up my backpack, resolved to leave. I'll walk out towards the sea, which isn't far from here. Nature will take care of me. I'm sure I'll be well looked after by Her.

I haul the rucksack onto my back and do up the strap around my waist. I'm not going to tell anyone I'm going, because they'll probably try to stop me. I'll just sneak out the way I came in. I make my way to the entrance and turn the handle but it doesn't open. *Damn.* It's locked.

A female member of staff rushes up to me.

'I'm just going out for a walk.' I've got a huge pack on, and it's obvious I'm checking out but I pretend anyway, just in case she buys it.

'I'm sorry, I can't let you out.'

'I'm here voluntarily so I should be allowed out.'

'I'm sorry. You're under observation for three days and I can't let you out until you've been seen by a doctor.' The woman is genuinely apologetic. I can tell she's anxious about doing her job properly and not being responsible for losing a patient on her watch.

'I'm so sorry. I totally understand and I don't want to get you into any trouble.' I have my hand on my heart, sincerely, but at the same time a rage is burning up through me. Remembering the Largactil scene with Joan, when she was dragged away for causing a fuss, I keep it pushed down, somewhere just below my chest, long enough to make my way quickly back to my room. As soon as I'm in there, I grab the pillow and scream into it, muffling the sound so as not to attract any attention. I don't want to be injected just because they're afraid of my anger.

Resigned to another adventure in this insane asylum, I unpack my stuff all over again and sit on the bed. I cross my legs and close my eyes, turning my attention inwards. Resting the tip of my tongue gently behind the top of my front teeth is like plugging into the mains and connects me to an internal circuit of energy flowing up my front and down my back. A buzzing feeling moves from the centre of my chest, out sideways in a loop, back to my heart and out the other way forming another circle. It keeps repeating this figure of eight. I turn my hands upwards, exposing my palms and then a Blake poem comes to me.

> To see a world in a grain of sand
> And a heaven in a wild flower
> Hold infinity in the palm of your hand
> And eternity in an hour

* * *

Every morning, just like Nelson Mandela did for twenty-seven years, I make my bed meticulously. It's not OCD, it's a feeling of reverence. I smooth out the sheets, which glide easily over the plastic mattress and I tuck them perfectly into each corner. I plump up the synthetic pillow in its starched cotton case, arranging it squarely at the top of the bed. Then I throw over the blankets, one at a time: beautiful, white, woven covers, with a knotted design that leaves tiny holes between the threads, like lace. I need at least three layers to block out the cold air. I like to snuggle down under the covers and burrow like an animal. These blankets haven't changed since I was first admitted, sixteen years ago.

Unlike Nelson Mandela, though, I don't read the newspapers. I watched him in a documentary once, carefully taking the corner and turning the page slowly and perfectly. He wasn't in any hurry. It was probably his only contact with the outside world. I prefer to keep away from big headlines. They send me off down a spiralling rabbit hole of fearful thoughts.

I clean my teeth, thoroughly, giving each individual tooth proper attention. I'm normally in a rush to get it done as quickly as possible, a chore that has to be ticked off my list. But today, and every day in this state, it's as if I'm doing it for the first time. I feel a tickly buzz in my head, the vibration from the electric toothbrush. I wash my face tenderly and delicately, enjoying the lather of the soap. Splashing water to get the suds off, I think about Ciaran.

Oh, Ciaran. I'm here again, in the psychiatric unit.

I pull the plug and the water gurgles his response as it goes down the plughole.

You should see the space I'm in!

He must be in quite a state with his wife divorcing him, but isn't it just like him to be so tit for tat?

Back in my room, way off in the distance, maybe a mile away, maybe more, I'm not sure, I hear the faint pounding of drums. It's like a calling to return home. I want to stamp around my room and howl to the spirits to come and work their magic in this place: to wake the staff up out of their delusional roles and to empower the patients out of their victimised states so they can live their lives to the full.

My door opens to a female member of staff.

'Emma. You've got visitors.'

'Who's here?'

'A couple of your friends.'

'Who?'

'I don't know.'

'I'm not going out there.' She ducks down making herself smaller, like an animal tiptoeing around a potential predator. Keeping her awareness on me, she moves across the tiny room to the chair, which she perches on.

'But your friends have come to see you,' she says softly.

'I'm not going out there if I don't know who's there.' I'm feeling a little paranoid and untrusting. I don't know what I'm expecting out there. I only go out of my room for meals and I've got used to being on my own in here, where it feels safe. The ward is full of dodgy-looking men who look threatening. One of them sits at the end of the women's corridor, like he's waiting for something. It unnerves me. Why the women's corridor? There's another bloke who looks like a drug dealer and always seems to be behind me in the queue for the canteen. He stands really tall and straight, and there's a violence in him that seems ready to burst out at the slightest provocation. His top two front teeth are missing so his incisors look like fangs. There's a dark hue coming off his face and he carries that intense expression of an addict.

It could be anyone out there pretending to be my friend.

The Polish nurse doesn't give up on me, gently nudging me to go out and see my visitors. I don't know whether to trust her. She's highly attuned to me, and flinches at the slightest of my gestures. She's obviously on hyper-alert but she's also empathetic and respectful.

'OK. I'll come and see who it is,' I relent, gathering up all the courage I can muster.

Angela and Nicky are waiting in the lobby with warm smiles on their faces. Angela puts her arm around me as we make our way down a curved corridor to a meeting room. The relief of her human touch is too much. I sob. I sound like an old lady I once saw in a Scandinavian film, suffering from dementia. She would spend her days lying in bed weeping a low quivering moan until her husband, with all the love in the world, put a pillow over her head. He couldn't bear her pain. The poor woman was probably just releasing old traumas, the dementia allowing her repressed pain to break through.

'Oh Emma,' Angela coos sympathetically, fuelling more sobbing from me. *She* doesn't need me to hide my emotions.

The room we go into is oppressive in its starkness. Nicky's face is tensed up while Angela, by contrast, is more open and tuned into me.

'I brought you my drum,' Angela says, handing me a hessian bag.

'Wow, thanks for lending it to me. I know how precious this is to you.' She made it herself with natural materials, carefully selected to suit her. Angela has the most beautiful voice and posture; she reminds me of a carved wooden Balinese puppet that my father brought back from a business trip. She has the same long neck and prominent nose.

'Is it pony skin?' I ask.

'No, it's made from deer skin.'

'What made me think it's pony skin? I keep wondering about it since I texted you to bring it.'

'That's so interesting. It *was* a choice between pony and deer, so perhaps you picked up on that.'

'It's weird in here. I don't like it,' I say looking around. They've brought me to the room I usually meet the psychiatrist in, and it's giving me the creeps.

They lean over me, their attention focused on my every move. Angela's ears twitch slightly whenever her eyebrows lift. She's like a fawn watching its mother, just in case she has to run. At the same time, she's like a doe ready to protect her offspring from danger: mother and baby all rolled into one. Nicky's anxious mothering has gone. She's very different to the Nicky who wept when I was taken off to hospital. She is distant, like she's split off somewhere else and the part of her that's here is on guard.

It's an awkward moment and they don't seem to know how to help me through it. My anxiety grows with their own increasingly concerned faces, which only leads to more fear in me, followed by more concern in them. We're caught in a mirroring loop: three highly sensitive people all feeding each other's fears.

I can't handle it and want to scream, like a pressure cooker that needs to be taken off the hob. I succumb to my basic flight instinct.

'This isn't working. I have to go back to my room.'

'Maybe it was a mistake to come,' Angela says, blaming herself. It wasn't a mistake. I clearly needed the human contact, but none of us is centred enough to handle it. I walk with them back to the entrance to the ward and leave them there, re-entering alone.

Back in my room, I take out the drum and look at it more closely. An owl feather dangles off the padded beater. I think about playing it but the mood has gone. I don't want to draw attention to myself. Everyone will think I'm crazier than they already do.

I have more visitors. This time I'm told who it is so I don't freak out. I exit the women's ward, my parents' smiling faces coming towards me as soon as they see me emerge. Mum opens her arms and squeezes me tightly. Dad isn't so emotional but hugs me more stiffly, in his usual way.

They think it's a good idea to take me to the beach in Torquay, which is nearby. I've never been, as it's quite urban, but I've been longing to get out of the hospital so I get my coat and follow them to their car.

'Your new flat is lovely, isn't it?' Mum says.

'Yeah. It's really spacious with the conservatory on the back.'

'It's good having the living room in there, isn't it? We've been watching the birds in the garden. Your neighbour's got a few budgies!'

'Yeah. I want to set them free but they're probably the only love in his life. His wife seems quite hard. Have you met them?'

'No. We met the new tenant that's upstairs in your old place though. She seems nice. She was very concerned about you, asking how you were.'

'She's a worrier.'

The beach is pebbly and not very wide as the tide is quite high. It's not that long either but we take our time walking along it. I like the shapes and patterns of the stones: aubergine, red, green, grey, and white lines swirl on them like marble. I pick up a few and walk up to the water's edge. I make three wishes silently in my head, one for each stone. Then I lob them in one at a time, enjoying the plopping sound.

'We just need to stop off at ASDA on the way back; we need to get some food in.'

'I can't go in a supermarket!'

'Don't worry. I'll be quick. You can stay in the car with Dad.'

The car park is busy. People are probably having their first shop after Christmas. Time goes slowly, waiting for Mum. Dad keeps watching me in his rear view mirror, checking I'm OK. Cars are constantly coming and going, revving their engines, starting up, reversing out, and pulling in.

Shame creeps through my body again, as if from nowhere. It's sticky, and cloying, and makes me squirm. Dad's eyes flash at me like he knows what's going on. Maybe it's written all over my face. I've no idea.

The best thing to do would be to get out of the car, go back to the beach, fill my pockets and walk right in. *Like Virginia Woolf did*, I think. Just as I reach for the door handle, Dad starts up the engine. He checks his mirror and looks at me before reversing out of the parking space. He drives very slowly to the entrance where Mum is waiting with the shopping. The forward motion of the vehicle pulls me out of my crippling inward spiral and within seconds the feeling has completely gone.

New Year's Eve comes and goes. I'm relieved there's no celebration to mark it on the ward as I'm still keeping away from the other patients. It feels like a healthy choice to look after myself. They spend most of their time smoking in the courtyard.

I notice on the activity board there's a minibus going to a pool in Newton Abbot. I let it be known that I'd like to go. A sporty-looking guy collects us in a minibus: me and two other patients. The male patient sits up front and rolls a cigarette, which he smokes with the window down. He talks non-stop, a little manically, but nothing sinister. The driver-cum-occupational-cum-therapist-cum-sportsman listens patiently, saying the odd word to let him know he's listening. The female patient sits in the back with me. She's wearing an electric blue puffa jacket and rolls herself a ciggie. She's not that interested in me. Not as much as I am in her.

'They've taken my daughter away.'

'Who have?'

'The authorities. She's gone off to Canada with her grandparents.'

'That must be hard. Why did they take her away from you?'

'They saw a video of me on the internet talking about having been abducted by aliens.'

'*Were* you abducted by aliens?'

'Yes. They took me to their laboratory and extracted all these samples from me. They had my daughter, too, and ran lots of tests on us both.'

'So what are you going to do about your daughter?'

'I'm going to go to Canada to get her back.'

I've not been to Newton Abbot pool before so I don't know my way around. It seems like quite a nice place. Better than the grimy Totnes one, anyhow. I follow the signs to the changing rooms. There are lots of children around. It's a long time since I've been to a public swim. I normally go to the lane swimming sessions so I can get my head down and do my lengths.

I don't feel self-conscious, so much as invaded. Every little sound and look that people make twangs somewhere inside me. My body is like a musical instrument being plucked and played by invisible hands. I have no energetic boundary between myself and anyone else. Like fabric that you stretch out, and if one part of it moves the whole cloth follows, because the threads are all connected.

I dive into the water, the sudden silence calming me. I stretch out my arms in a breaststroke, swimming a whole length underwater, emerging on the surface to take a sharp breath. The din of kids playing is a sudden onslaught to my ears, like opening the door to a noisy room. I close it again, ducking down and swimming beneath them all.

It's too busy to do my usual lengths. I'd have to keep weaving in and out of people. If I stay underwater I can swim deep enough to get a clear run. It's quieter, too. I'm like a shark in the deep, watching legs kicking above me.

It's tiring holding my breath and I'm feeling quite weak so I don't stay in the pool for very long. When the rest of them have finished, we all pile back into the minibus. The way back is more peaceful, the swimming having done everyone the world of good.

'You're a good swimmer,' the driver/chaperone etc. compliments me.

'I usually swim every day. Forty lengths of a twenty-five metre pool.'

'A kilometre. That's pretty good.'

'It helps me sleep. It burns off excess energy and keeps me fit. I love it. I'm a water baby.'

When we get back to the psychiatric ward, I head straight for my room.

CHAPTER THIRTY

Voices

Another drive home from another hospital where I've only been for a week this time. Not losing my ego has enabled me to stay in this world, the one that psychiatrists think is the real one. Plus having parents who negotiate my release and are happy to take care of me, means I'm let out quickly.

Julie Andrews is on the radio and I comment that thinking about your favourite things is a rather outdated coping strategy, as it doesn't actually deal with the darker stuff. Singing along, I feel like the Dame herself, and Mum joins in. When we get to the 'dog bites' part, we turn to each other and hiss out the word 'bites', hamming it up like we're on stage. My singing voice always sounds better in my episodes. I don't know why. It might be because my throat is less tense, or it might just be my hearing that's more finely tuned. Who cares? It sends me off into memories of being in the local pantomime as a kid. I loved the camaraderie and entertaining people. Mum used to enjoy being on stage, too. Until Dad put a stop to it. Well, that's how the story goes, anyway.

'You should go on stage,' I say to Mum.

'Rubbish.'

'You once told me that Dad forbade it.'

'Yes. I'd got a part in a play, but I got pregnant.'

'I didn't forbid you!' Dad butts in. Perhaps Mum is remembering it wrong.

'It's too late now, anyway. I'm too old. *You* should go on stage,' Mum says, taking the attention off herself.

'I might. I did love it, but I get too much stage fright now.'

Musical interlude over, I enjoy the rest of the ride home, feeling each car passing by, and whether it's good energy or bad energy: raindrops on roses, or dog bites and bee stings.

It's so good to get home where I can potter around, make healthy meals, and listen to the radio. I have it on as a soundtrack to my cooking. Like the classic Morecambe and Wise breakfast sketch, where they dance around the kitchen to the striptease tune, I move around to the music. Taking a side step and sliding my other foot to join it, tango-like, I open a cupboard door. Even when the radio is switched off, I still feel the pulsing of life taking me as its partner. My every move is a dance, connected through the fabric of space, to the rhythm of the universe.

* * *

Melissa has an amazing summerhouse that she had built where their rather large old garage used to be. Melissa and Tim live in a farmhouse with a few acres of land where Tim grows organic vegetables. They also have a collection of animals to keep their only daughter Katie company: a couple of cows, a couple of tortoises, a couple of guinea pigs, a couple of dogs, a cat, and a snake. It's like Noah's Ark. I love spending time there and now that Melissa is no longer a client of mine, I've developed a great friendship with her. She has spared no expense in converting the garage into the most beautiful, calm, welcoming space.

The friends that make up my care team are meeting there to air their grievances about looking after me. I wonder what they have to say but neither Melissa nor I want to join them. Instead she picks me up in her white Toyota Prius and drives us to the beach. It's a blustery January day and a coast walk will clear out the cobwebs.

I take the passenger's seat with Millie, their longhaired Jack Russell next to my feet in the footwell, avoiding the worst of her travel sickness. Chloe, their beautiful velvety grey whippet hogs the back seat, like the princess she is, in a class of her own. I'm finely tuned into the energy around me: the rhythm and pace of the natural environment and I can tell, by the way Melissa is driving, that she is too.

'Your driving is great. You're really tuned in.'

'You're so present. I've never seen you so present before.' I'm glad she notices. It's not something the mental health service pays any attention to.

Trying to get to the beach on this bit of South Devon coastline involves navigating narrow country lanes with high hedges. There's never much room and the passing places are essential. One lone female rider is all we see, holding tight to her reins and fussing nervously on her horse, who is reflecting her anxiety right back to her. Melissa slows down to a respectful speed so as not to spook the animal and it relaxes a little as it senses the change in our approach. The woman, though, is all a-fluster and pulls harder on the reins, making the horse tighten up again in response. She gestures with her hands for us to slow down even though we're going well below the speed limit.

'She doesn't realise we're in tune with the universe, does she?' Melissa laughs.

'No and the horse is fine with us,' I reply. 'It's her that's freaking it out.' We pass slowly, giving them a wide berth.

Melissa parks in a small car park overlooking Bigbury Beach. A man with a surfboard on his roof rack stands looking out to sea and Mel goes over to chat to him. I stay back, uncomfortable with any social interaction involving strangers. I want to check him out, because he's quite good-looking, but can't find the courage, so I wait for Mel to return.

The wind is dramatic by the sea and it's blowing from all directions. We head west along the coast path letting the dogs tear off in the vast open fields. When we reach a clifftop I comment on the feeling I'm getting in my body.

'Make a sound.' Melissa suggests so I try to put a note to the strange sensation quivering through me.

'*Ahhhhhhhhhh.*' It's quite high-pitched, like an alarm call. I'm not sure what's making me feel so distressed. Perhaps it's just the crazy wind agitating me.

Millie and Chloe have done their usual disappearing act, no doubt chasing some poor wild creature.

'Millie! Chloe!' Melissa yells, trying to call them back to us but there's no sign of them.

'I've found if I put my attention into my womb and psychically call them from there, they return within two minutes,' I explain. I often walk these dogs for Mel when I dog-sit for her and I've got to know their ways. They can disappear off for hours sometimes. I drop into my lower belly and intentionally connect to Chloe to tell her to come back. Sure enough within a minute Millie's head is bobbing through the grass and Chloe is galloping along not far behind.

'It works every time!' I exclaim.

A dead rabbit is sticking out from either side of Chloe's mouth and she holds it on the ground by Melissa, as if offering her a gift. I burst out laughing, finding it hilarious for some unfathomable reason. Millie tries to take the poor bunny off Chloe but Chloe is not going to give it up. A tug of war ensues, causing Mel to shout at them to stop. I'm in fits of laughter, not holding back. It's the look on Chloe's face that's tickling me. In her expression I can see a kind of yeah what, pretend innocence. Mel takes hold of Millie to pull her away, knowing from experience that they don't know when to stop. They are surprisingly evenly matched, even though there's a huge difference in size between them. Melissa succeeds in separating them and insists Chloe drop the kill. Reluctantly, Chloe opens her mouth and dumps the dead rabbit on the ground.

* * *

Ciaran emails me to tell me he's got together with someone who I worked with on the Transition film. It happened three months ago. After a quick calculation I figure out it must have been just before the divorce was finalised. It's brought up a lot of emotions that I've somehow bypassed until now.

When I see our car parked down the road, I want to slash the tyres and scratch the paintwork but I know it won't make me feel any better. Sometimes it sits there overnight and I imagine he's staying at *her* house. Why else would it be there for so long? Every time I see it I go through the same battle, picturing me running the key along the side of it and stabbing the wheels. Now, I only have to see any old pale blue Ford Focus to feel the anger rising. It's a conditioned response, the shape and colour triggering a traumatised state in me.

I realise I don't have to keep putting myself through the stress of it so ask Ciaran not to park on my street any more. At first he says there isn't anywhere else so I find another lane for him that doesn't have any parking restrictions.

It feels good asking for some consideration. Learning to assert myself, instead of being a doormat, I'm surprised by the uplifting effect it has on me. It feels liberating and empowering to know how much more responsible I am for how I feel than I'd previously imagined.

Ciaran and I had some lovely times together. It was mostly cosy and supportive. He cheered me on with my filming achievements and I celebrated his writing and his work with young offenders. We were a great team. He helped with the cleaning without being asked and did his fair share of shopping and cooking. He was easy to live with and I cared deeply for him as he did for me. But we were never meant to be together as man and wife. We were friends not lovers and neither of us did anything wrong to cause our marriage to break down. We settled for each other because it felt good but it wasn't really a sexual relationship. I was his soul sister not his soul mate.

Once I've got used to the idea of him moving on, I make peace with it. I admit to myself that I don't actually want to be with him anyway, so why shouldn't he be happy with someone else? I've been holding out for Ciaran to tell me I'm the woman for him and that he doesn't want to be without me but I haven't actually asked myself whether he's the man for me. That's the more relevant question. Now I'm free to find the right man for me, I'm going to have a lot of fun looking.

* * *

I was first introduced to Katie through a mutual friend on Facebook. She's sparkly-eyed with a white-blonde cropped haircut and pointy ears, like a pixie in human form. She had a profound awakening a few years ago and feared she was going crazy. She was working in mental health services at the time and knew not to mention it to anyone at work because she wanted her experiences to be validated rather than pathologised. She left her job and is now co-ordinating a training programme introducing Open Dialogue into the NHS.

Open Dialogue is a new form of psychiatric care that was developed in Finland, a country that used to have the worst statistics for schizophrenia in Europe but now has the best. Tornio, a region in Western Lapland, actually scrapped their entire psychiatric system and started again, it was that bad. A bunch of progressive family therapists got together and asked themselves how they could do it better. Gradually they developed a system based on some key principles: a belief in the ability of a person to get well; and an understanding that mental health issues are a systemic problem that results from the breakdown of social relationships, and not because there is something inherently wrong with one individual. A team is allocated to the person at the centre of concern (they're not called a patient) who has to be seen within twenty-four hours. That same team then stays with them for the whole course of treatment. The person at the centre of concern chooses their social network to attend regular meetings. The length and regularity of these meetings is decided by the family members themselves. There is no diagnosis but instead a focus on dialogue, encouraging everybody's voice to be heard. Medication is kept to a minimum and discussed with everyone, and no discussions are to take place without the people present. It's so radical that it is hard for Western-trained medics to comprehend how it could work, they're so programmed by the broken-brain theory.

When I get an email from Katie, tentatively wondering if I'd be interested in filming the course for online learning, I practically bite her hand off. They can't pay very much and she's a little embarrassed asking me, but I assure her it's a subject close to my heart so I don't mind. I find it fitting that the NHS will be giving me money to film what I hope will mark a turning point in the psychiatric system. My professional life has finally come together with my personal one: Green Lane Films meets *My Beautiful Psychosis*.

Every level of mental health professional is attending the course: psychiatrists, social workers, psychotherapists, nurses, carers, consultants, and even a chaplain. It's so different from how they're used to working, it's bringing up a lot of resistance, concerns, questions, and emotions.

'I feel really guilty for the kind of care we've been providing all these years. Now I'm wondering what the hell all my medical training was for,' one brave consultant admits.

It's an intense week and I haven't really thought about the emotional impact it would have on me. The job I've got to do is really straightforward. I just have to record all the sessions and put them online so that those who miss any can catch up. It's not a creative challenge, which is just as well because it's bringing up loads of undigested stuff I've had to swallow over the years. Feelings I chose to hide in order to play the system are resurfacing. I make sure to check in with myself daily and let these emotions out privately so it doesn't interfere with my work. Every morning I cry my way through painful memories. An occasional tear escapes while I'm filming but only Katie notices. She always looks at me at particularly poignant moments, because she's invariably welling up too.

The guy who's running the course, Dr Russell Razzaque, is a consultant psychiatrist who wrote a book called *Breaking Down Is Waking Up*.

Russell got into all of this because someone recommended a retreat to help him de-stress. He went to a place not far from Totnes called Gaia House, which is a Buddhist centre, and he had no idea he was going to have to spend the whole weekend in silence. Through mindfulness, he discovered that his mind was as crazy with thoughts as any of his manic patients. He wasn't looking for a spiritual fix—in fact he was an atheist—but what he found, when his mind finally stopped for a few moments, was a profound feeling of paradox: that he was nothing and everything at the same time. It was not unlike some of the states that his psychotic patients described. After that, he never quite saw them in the same way again. He now believes that every psychosis carries the potential for transformation, and to heavily medicate people is to close them down, miss an amazing opportunity, and do them a great disservice. I wish this guy had been my doctor. I'm the founding member of the Russell Razzaque Fan Club.

I also believe psychosis has much potential for healing and though this idea is not new, it has been considered controversial, responded to with guffaws and dismissals. Since at least the time of Carl Jung, and perhaps more famously R. D. Laing, clinicians and individuals with lived experience have been discussing the transformative power of psychosis.

I hook up with Russell over meal times to get to know him a little more. I'm impressed with the diplomacy he's had to use to get Open Dialogue into the NHS. He's managed to convince chief executives to take money out of severely compromised frontline services to pay for training. To be putting forward such an alternative approach in a system that's so dependent on the pharmaceutical industry takes guts—and all this in the midst of austerity.

'One of the student psychiatrists said that you were very courageous, Russell. But I wonder. Courage is only necessary when you're afraid and you don't seem scared at all. But maybe I'm wrong. Are you?' I ask him one morning at breakfast.

'I'm terrified. Sometimes I wake up in a sweat and wonder what the hell I'm doing.'

'Well, you hide it well; you seem so calm and relaxed.'

'That's all the mindfulness training.' Russell pauses before continuing, 'Katie tells me you have lived experience. There's an opportunity at the end of the week for people to share whatever they like. It would be great if you were to introduce yourself and say something. I think it would be good for people to hear what you have to say.'

'Thanks, Russell. I really feel like I need to do that. I'm finding it quite frustrating not being able to join in from behind the camera.'

There's lots I want to say. I write down in my notebook all that's bubbling up. It takes me a few days to get past the bitterness. By the end of the week I have ten pages of scribblings. Each page is a reworking, to get it absolutely right. I don't want to blow this opportunity. I need to say something that will have an impact, not shy away from my truth, but respect that they're on a difficult journey and probably need some encouragement to stick at it.

The course participants are blown away by how much their guinea-pig families have been opening up during Open Dialogue meetings. It's typical for a family member to say things they've never said to anyone else before. That's what happens when you create a safe space where you listen instead of label. I can't help thinking it's not rocket science, and am pissed off they never bothered to get to know their patients before.

Some of them are quite resistant, wanting to know the theory behind it, satisfying their thinking minds rather than feeling the wisdom of it through their hearts, which I find really annoying. But I remember the undoing I had to go through when I first learnt shiatsu. I wanted to know how it all worked before I would trust it. This is no different. It's been drilled into them that mental illness is a brain chemical imbalance that requires medication, so no wonder it's hard to get their heads around the idea that doing nothing is more effective. What they don't realise is that listening with an empty mind and an open heart is not doing nothing. It's probably the hardest thing to be able to do if you've been educated in a system that rewards you for being knowledgeable and clever.

I think the word 'mental' health is misleading. I'm convinced that it's our emotional health that causes the disturbances in brain function. For example, intense fear plus low self-esteem results in paranoia. Paranoia is considered a symptom, but I think it is fear projected out onto the world.

In Western cultures, someone describing unusual experiences (for example auditory or visual hallucinations) is likely to be perceived as harbouring some internal biochemical imbalance that requires treatment with medication. The person already struggling with these unusual experiences is forced to choose between either accepting this view, or dismissing it and risking coercion into unwanted treatment or withdrawal of support. The parallel with the medieval witch-hunts is striking. If you admit you're a witch, you'll be burnt or hanged. If you deny it, you'll be put through a test you can't win, one in which your innocence will be proved by your death. Something happened to me when I was faced with this dilemma myself. I felt like I was seeing the world as it really was for the first time but the doctors saw me as deluded. I had to play their game because if I insisted on my reality being the true one then that only proved my insanity. I felt a split happen in my head as I tried to navigate a lose-lose situation. It damaged my trust and faith in the medical model.

What I needed was a judgement-free curiosity about my experience so that it was safe to share what was going on inside me. I avoided telling people what was really happening because of how it was perceived, even to the extreme of becoming mute. I was going through some disturbing experiences, my psyche exploring much undigested psychological material, and I needed help. Instead of integrating all of these parts of myself, I had to put them on hold and go into survival mode, to survive the psychiatric system.

It's not possible to medicate away aspects of myself that need attending to. That only adds further to the pushing away of it all. What you resist persists, right? The only way through is actually facing it and making friends with these lost parts of myself, learning to listen to and accept and love even the darkest recesses of my psyche.

What if we took individuals who are experiencing emotional crises called 'psychosis' and offered them safe spaces of respite? What if the therapist was more of a guide and support, allowing the person to go through their experience and help them to make meaning from it? What if interventions were based on respect for the psychotic experience and all it represents, and focused on ensuring that the person feels safe, supported, heard, and understood? What if people who had gone through the experience themselves were to teach others how to navigate it, or train mental health professionals to better care for them?

Not having all the answers, not making a diagnosis or deciding on an appropriate prescription is making some of the participants feel impotent. That might be something they've been trying to avoid feeling their entire lives: a core wound driving them on to be the big saviour. Believing that their patients actually have the power within to heal themselves is a 180 degree turn-around in their thinking.

I have to remind myself that these are the good guys. These are the ones who are unhappy with the system as it is and care enough to try something new. Open Dialogue is a beacon of hope that I believe has the potential to transform our entire relationship to mental health. It acknowledges the importance of relationships and sees mental distress as a sign that they have broken down in some way. The person who is supposedly ill is merely expressing the sickness in the family, like the canary in the coalmine. Being more sensitive, they simply feel the damage that the dysfunctional family dynamics are causing. Shouldn't we be rewarding people for that?

I've come to realise that I am sensitive and need to respect this sensitivity. I don't and can't filter out the world as other people do. I feel deeply all that's happening, because we're interconnected, and I can't ignore that. I see the beauty and love, but also the pain and damage. Sometimes I want to be able to switch it all off and be normal like everyone else. But going into the fire has purified me. It has burnt away a lot of stuff that I don't need to carry around any more.

It's the closing session, a goldfish bowl, where a circle of chairs is placed in the centre of the room for whoever wishes to say something. The first round of people sit down and share their thoughts about the week. Is this the moment that Russell was referring to? Is he going to introduce me or do I just take a seat when one becomes available? I let the others do the talking and decide not to dominate with my probably unwelcome opinion.

'It's nearly five o'clock now so we'll have to make this the last round,' Russell says as he sits in one of the chairs. The other teachers stand up and join him: Mark Hopfenberg, who has come from Norway, has been teaching Open Dialogue for years; and Val, a family therapist from Yorkshire. I know Val won't like what I have to say. I saw her face flush and her eyes flash when she overhead me talking about spiritual stuff over lunch one day. She looked like she wanted to put her hand over my mouth because I was saying something forbidden. I didn't really understand it at the time but Katie says that Val is a solid Yorkshire lass with no time for any wishy-washy stuff.

Mark shares how privileged he feels to be working in this way and is so moved he looks like he's going to break down. I don't really listen to Val because I can't help staring at the empty seat next to her. A thought keeps coming into my head and it won't go away.

Sit in the chair. Sit in the chair. Sit in the chair.

Russell takes the floor, which means my window of opportunity is about to close. With a powerful force coursing through me, I take the place between him and Val. When Russell has finished, I ignore my blind panic and open my mouth.

'It looks like I'm going to get the last word.' I pause for laughter. 'You talk about Open Dialogue being about allowing all the voices to be heard. Well, I need to bring a voice into the room, which is never normally permitted within the psychiatric system. It's a voice that gets pathologised because you all think it's not real. The voice of spirit.

'It's no accident that I am the person behind the camera. I had my first episode in 1996 and if there had been Open Dialogue then, my life would have been very different. Maybe I wouldn't have gone on to have six more episodes.

'When I had my first meeting with the consultants, I asked them what had happened to me. I thought I had had some kind of awakening. I remember their words exactly. "As far as we can tell, you've had some kind of psychotic episode." I was devastated to hear that and I burst into tears. There weren't even any tissues in the room. They only asked me one question. All they wanted to know was whether I had heard voices. When I said I had they made a note, satisfied that I'd confirmed their diagnosis. But if they'd asked me about the voice, like you probably would have done in an Open Dialogue meeting, if they'd bothered to include the voice instead of pathologising it, they would have discovered that it was the most angelic voice I had ever heard. "You are beautiful," it said. And it helped me in my hour of deepest need.

'So I want to thank spirit for bringing me here and for all that's happening. You've got your work cut out for you but don't ever doubt the importance of what you're all doing here. You're changing lives.' Then I raise my hands up to the sky, acknowledging a force that's way beyond me and my terrified little ego. 'Thank you.'

The room erupts in applause and Val is the first to open her arms, with tears in her eyes, and hug me.

And nobody thinks I'm crazy.

AFTERWORD

My mum often says, 'It'll be alright in the end so if it's not alright, it's not the end.' I was hoping to end this book by saying I no longer have episodes. I imagined I'd share my secret as to how I've achieved that. But I can't. I've had four more since number seven, making a total of eleven, to date. Each one I think is going to be the last. I was under the impression that as long as I didn't do any spiritual practices, workshops, residentials, retreats, or anything like that, I would be OK. But other stressful life circumstances have also set me off.

Some will conclude it's because I have a condition called bipolar or schizophrenia, a brain chemical imbalance and that's that. But I don't believe that. Sure, it would mean I am not responsible but it also disempowers me. It also means a lifelong prescription of soul-deadening medication. This might be ok for some, but it's not ok with me. The brain chemical imbalance theory turns out to be a story anyway, made up by the pharmaceutical industry and has never been proved. This perspective, held by the current psychiatric profession, has meant that no one has ever asked me what I was actually experiencing, beyond the symptoms. Nobody reached in, as a human being, to communicate with me and help me through my distress. If psychosis is a result of

273

relationships breaking down, as Open Dialogue principles suggest, then this only served to worsen the problem.

Having filmed Open Dialogue training for over two years, I feel for those working in the mental health services. They are in crisis and caught in a vicious circle: they don't understand enough about psychosis—so no one is trained to help properly—so people don't get the help they need—so there's increasing numbers of people who need help—but they don't understand enough about psychosis—so no one is trained to help properly—so they don't get the help they need—so there's increasing numbers of people who need help—and so it goes on. We need to break this cycle and I believe that Open Dialogue will do just that.

I've met many people through the Spiritual Crisis Network who emphasise the spiritual angle. It certainly validated many of my own experiences. But it feels oversimplifying to say that I'm having a spiritual awakening that is happening too quickly and too intensely. After all, spiritual awakenings are immediate and powerful by nature. No, something is definitely amiss and I want to get to the bottom of it.

I've come to the conclusion that I'm sensitive. When I was a baby, just six weeks old, the smallpox vaccine actually gave me cowpox. But I think I am also susceptible because of childhood sexual abuse. I've learnt to dissociate, as a defence mechanism, to cope with a traumatic situation, which I experience as being catapulted into other realms. I don't think I'm having a spiritual awakening so much as escaping into the spiritual dimension. The medical profession call these hallucinations but many people believe these realms exist, including me.

I think it's helpful to look at psychosis as a process of finding wholeness. The disintegration of the ego is a doorway through which the unconscious can be made conscious. The stuff that comes up can be seen as undigested psychological material that needs processing and integrating. It wants to be known. Not exploring the themes that come up is a missed opportunity. If we simply label it delusional and hallucinatory then we devalue it and, worse still, see it as a sign of illness.

I like William Blake's words in *The Marriage of Heaven and Hell*:

'If the doors of perception were cleansed every thing would appear to man as it is, infinite. For man has closed himself up, till he sees all things thro' narrow chinks of his cavern.'

We have evolved to perceive the world within a certain limited human range, one that favours optimum functioning to ensure survival and reproduction. But our brains are capable of perceiving more. I've been catapulted through those doors of perception. The question I am now asking is not whether it is real or hallucinatory but whether I want to close it or not. And if so, can I find the key?

But that's a whole other story.

ACKNOWLEDGEMENTS

Deep gratitude to Tom Petherick for allowing me to write in his shepherd's hut and not judging me when I hardly wrote a thing. A big thank you to Elizabeth Presland, my first reader, who didn't think I was crazy for seeing ancestral spirits. Much appreciation to Elizabeth Diamond, my first critic, for pointing out where my writing needed improving in the early stages. A heartfelt thanks to all those lovely people in the Totnes Writing Group who listened to me reading out extracts and encouraged me when I was feeling vulnerable. Thank you, thank you, thank you Nick Palmer for your help with formatting and producing the audiobook. A big thank you to my editor, Victoria Roddam, for believing in my manuscript and showing me what I still needed to do when I thought I had finished. To all my friends who have taken the greatest care of me—Anna, Conrad, Oli, Jeanne, Wendy, Diane, Boe, Sophy, Kamini, Agata, Aisla, Richenda, Beccy, Hannah, Alexandra, Toni, Cath, Netha, Sarah, Ruth and Sho—eternal thanks. You treated me with the utmost respect and didn't freak out when I was behaving rather strangely. And the deepest gratitude to Caspar for giving it his all. Also a massive thank you to Donovan who did the work that ten women couldn't to keep me out of hospital and then shone his light to help me out of the darkness. Last but not least, I give a deep bow to my family (particularly my parents) who are always there, travelling halfway around the world to make sure I'm OK. I am very lucky to have you. Not everyone is privileged enough to have a safe place to convalesce.

THANKS TO ALL THOSE WHO KINDLY DONATED
TO THE CROWDFUNDING CAMPAIGN

Maria Gatenby-Roberts, Nick Palmer, Jorgo De Groof, Graham Pirnie, Lucy Gatward, Kamini Gupta, Zanna Markillie, Peter Johnston, Tazeem Moledina, John Green, Kitty de Bruin, Johanna Ryder, Margaret and Malcolm Goude, Max Velmans, Anne and Pat O'Mara, Verran Townsend, Sara Haq, Sarah Melia, Phil Borges (Crazywise), Phillip Milman, Jilah Bakhshayesh, Dan Davies, Michelle Hobart, Joy Prater, and Nicola Ruane.

ABOUT THE AUTHOR

Emma Goude is an international award winning documentary filmmaker emerging from behind the camera to tell her own story. She has written *My Beautiful Psychosis* to help change the perception of psychosis as a debilitating illness. She hopes that sharing her story will inspire others, improve attitudes, and ultimately contribute to a better system of care. She is currently living in Buenos Aires where she is following her passion for dancing tango.

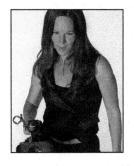

For more information please visit www.emmagoude.com